ESSENCE
OF
MATERIA MEDICA

by
GEORGE VITHOULKAS

Author of

- Additions of Kent's Repertory of the Homoeopathic Materia Medica
- Materia Medica Viva (**12** Vols.)
- Talks on Classical Homoeopathy
- The Science of Homeopathy

B. Jain Publishers (P) Ltd.

USA — Europe — India

ESSENCE OF MATERIA MEDICA

First Edition: 1988
Second Edition: 1990
17th Impression: 2014

Note from the Publishers
Any information given in this book is not intended to be taken as a replacement for medical advice. Any person with a condition requiring medical attention should consult a qualified practitioner or therapist.

All rights reserved. No part of this book may be reproduced, stored in a retrieval system or transmitted, in any form or by any means, mechanical, photocopying, recording or otherwise, without any prior written permission of the publisher.

© with the publisher

Published by Kuldeep Jain for
B. JAIN PUBLISHERS (P) LTD.
An ISO 9001 : 2000 Certified Company
1921/10, Chuna Mandi, Paharganj, New Delhi 110 055 (INDIA)
Tel.: +91-11-4567 1000 • Fax: +91-11-4567 1010
Email: info@bjain.com • Website: www.bjain.com

Printed in India by
J. J. Offset Printers

ISBN: 978-81-319-0201-1

Publisher's Note to the Second Edition

The "Essence of Materia Medica" had to be published, in a hurry, as soon as possible after the first Indian edition of George Vithoulkas's popular book: "Homoeopathy = Medicine of the New Man" came out, since it was a sort of a sequel to its appendix, wherein the essences of four homoeopathic polychrests - Nux-v., Lyc., Nat-m, and Phos. - were printed. So the bare text appeared in the first edition.

This second edition has been prepared with the text freed from the errors that the first one carried and an index of remedies added. It is expected that this index will facilitate understanding of the fine differences in the symptomatology of the remedies answering the same rubric in the repertory, thus help pick up the right remedy for the case in hand.

In the text abbreviations instead of the full names of the remedies has been uniformly used for the sake of uniformity and brevity. The List of "Remedies and their abbreviations" appearing on H. Barthel's SYNTHETIC REPERTORY has been adhered to for this purpose.

It will be evident to the reader that GV has drawn heavily from Kent, mainly his lectures on "Homoeopathic Materia Medica" and his "Repertory" — the two of his famous trio. While, acknowledging these quotes, GV takes the trouble to point out where his own experience differed from that of the great Master.

Further in order to understand GV, it would be necessary to have access to his own Opus magnum: "Science of Homoeopathy", whose pages may further throw light on his explanations and speculations as to how or why a remedy was chosen, etc.

The treatment of the fiftyone remedies in this volume is an illustration of what is meant by carrying the Materia Medica in one's head for use at the beside! It is hoped in this improved edition, this book will prove on befitting companion to the author's other work which Dr. BILL GRAY of USA has called "a landmark work" and help further comprehension of the "seemingly miraculous method" of cure!

CONTENTS

	Publisher's Note	i
1.	AETHUSA CYNAPIUM (*aeth.*)	1
2.	AGARICUS MUSCARIUS (*agar.*)	2
3.	AGNUS CASTUS (*agn.*)	3
4.	ALUMINA (*alum.*)	5
5.	ARGENTUM NITRICUM (*arg-n.*)	10
6.	ARSENICUM ALBUM (*ars.*)	14
7.	AURUM FOLIATUM (*aur.*)	21
8.	BARYTA CARBONICA (*bar-c.*)	26
9.	BISMUTHUM SUBNITRICUM (*bism.*)	30
10.	BRYONIA (*bry.*)	32
11.	CALCAREA CARBONICA (*calc.*)	37
12.	CALCAREA PHOSPHORICA (*calc-p.*)	42
13.	CANNABIS INDICA (*cann-i.*)	47
14.	CAPSICUM ANNUUM (*caps.*)	52
15.	CAUSTICUM HAHNEMANNI (*caust.*)	54
16.	CARBO VEGETABILIS (*carb-v.*)	59
17.	CHELIDONIUM MAJUS (*chel.*)	64
18.	DULCAMARA (*dulc.*)	68
19.	FLUORICUM ACIDUM (*fl-ac.*)	72
20.	GRAPHITES NATURALIS (*graph.*)	74
21.	GRATIOLA OFFICINALIS (*grat.*)	79
22.	HEPAR SULPHURIS CALCAREUM (*hep.*)	80
23.	HYDROPHOBINUM LYSSINUM (*lyss.*)	83
24.	HYOSCYAMUS NIGER (*hyos.*)	85
25.	IGNATIA AMARA (*ign.*) (first version)	88
26.	IGNATIA AMARA (*ign.*) (second version)	91
27.	KALI BICHROMICUM (*kali-bi.*)	94
28.	KALI CARBONICUM (*kali-c.*)	99
29.	LACHESIS MUTA (*lach.*)	105
30.	LYCOPODIUM CLAVATUM (*lyc.*)	108
31.	MAGNESIA MURIATICA (*mag-m.*)	113
32.	MEDORRHINUM (*med.*)	117
33.	MERCURIUS SOLUBILIS (*merc.*)	123

34.	NATRUM MURIATICUM (nat-m.)	130
35.	NITRIC ACID (nit-ac.)	138
36.	NUX VOMICA (nux-v.)	143
37.	PHOSPHORICUM ACIDUM (ph-ac.)	150
38.	PHOSPHORUS (phos.)	155
39.	PLATINUM METALLICUM (plat.)	160
40.	PLUMBUM MATALLICUM (plb.)	165
41.	PULSATILLA PRATENSIS (puls.)	171
42.	RHUS TOXICODENDRON (Rhus-t.)	173
43.	SEPIA SUCCUS (sep.) (FIRST VERSION)	175
44.	SEPIA SUCCUS (sep.) (SECOND VERSION)	178
45.	SILICA (sil.)	180
46.	STANNUM METALLICUM (stann.)	184
47.	STAPHYSAGRIA (staph.)	188
48.	STRAMONIUM (stram.)	194
49.	SYPHILINUM (syph.)	198
50.	TARENTULA HISPANICA (tarent.)	200
51.	THUJA OCCIDENTALIS (thuj.)	204
52.	TUBERCULINUM BOVINUM KENT (tub.)	209
53.	VERATRUM ALBUM (verat.)	212
54.	INDEX OF REMEDIES	214

AETHUSA CYNAPIUM (*aeth.*)

The Chronic Type

— Individuals who feel apart.
— Strong emotions but do not express them easily.
— Moved to tears but do not actually cry—emotions felt inside (Unlike Ignatia—moved to tears but constricted at throat so doesn't cry).
— Own emotional world—very intense.
— Live happily by themselves, but also enjoy company.
— Talk to themselves.

Sleep

— Intensity comes out in sleep—sleepwalks.
— Deep sleep on either left or right side.
— Salivate during sleep.
— "FEAR of closing eyes lest should never wake."—Kent.
— < darkness—do not like darkness—fear will not wake up again. Feel as if suffocating from darkness—have to open window, (Lachesis, Grindelia).
— Cannot control the breathing—have to get up, (Ignatia—fear will never sleep again).
— Fear of not waking up after an operation.

EXTRA NOTES

— Crazy for animals, cats and dogs etc—look after them with unnatural passion.
— Talk to animals when don't talk to people.
— Great irritability.
— P.M.T.—tremendous build up, headache, feel rotten two days before and days 1 and 2, then relax and libido increases immediately after menses.—Fear of losing a loved one is unbearable.
— Sudden redness in face with a wild look, and drawing feeling in face before or during menopause.
— Deep furrows in face in sick cases—look near death, look very old.

- Eruption on tip of nose, or between nostrils, or even in nostrils—recurrent (eczema or herpes etc.)
- < HEAT, ESPECIALLY SUMMER.
- Yellowish leucorrhoea which stains linen.
- Distension of abdomen when irritated, or if eat more than usual —sometimes have to induce vomiting to >.
- Craves cheese, FARINACEOUS food, salt.
- Averse : fruits.

AGARICUS MUSCARIUS (*agar.*)

The Mental/Emotional Picture

- Anxiety about health—will drive you crazy with it (Nit. ac, Ars, Phos, Kali ars.)
- Don't necessarily have the physical symptoms of Agaricus.
- Find something to suffer about: become anxious about some little thing, then it builds up and they become pessimistic. Finally, they don't want to live and go to doctor—the doctor's slightest suggestions are blown up in their minds, e.g. if doctor suggests a mammography they will have a fear of cancer for the rest of their lives.
- They cry ++ and are anxious and drive you mad.
- Sometimes ANXIETY state changes to a tremendous EUPHORIA, which they recognise is not quite healthy despite the euphoria, and so revert to anxiety.
- Out of the body experiences — feel well when come out of the body (Cann. ind. find it a terrifying experience).
- An element of spookiness about these people.
- Think about dead people.
- Can't sleep in certain beds because they look like coffins, or can't have sex in certain beds for this reason.
- Fear of cancer, but don't think they are going to die. They are always meeting or hearing of people who have cancer, like to help dying people.
- Aversion to eggs.
- Desires salt + nil else especially.
- < HEAT
- Hypochondriacal anxiety.

AGNUS CASTUS (*agn.*)

Agnus castus is a remedy which I believe will be increasingly needed in our modern societies, especially by the younger generation. It is indicated after a lot of abuses common among young people—sexual excesses, the use of psychoactive drugs, loss of sleep, sporadic nutrition, etc. Such people have been easily excitable, and engaged in many of these activities very intensely over a relatively brief period of time. Then they become pale, anaemic, low in energy, absent-minded etc.

Eventually these people begin to realize that their whole constitution is breaking down. They develop the fear that within a few years or a few months they are going to die. They feel they have over-exerted and dissipated their life energies to the point that their whole system has become rotten.

Such people reach a stage in which they are unable to concentrate any more on their studies, their daily tasks etc. They experience sexual impotency, and they become very preoccupied with this problem. They become convinced that they are about to have a nervous breakdown, or that their vital organs are about to collapse.

This concern becomes so great in Agnus castus that these people develop an anxiety about health which is almost hypochondriacal.

— voluptuous fantasies without erection, and finally into complete loss of sexual desire.

It also happens that the *Agnus* castus patient breaks down in another way: he sometimes feels that he is worthless, that he is absolutely useless in the world. And then, at other times, he feels that he is a very great man, that he is something quite special. These states then alternate with each other.

Women also may need *Agnus castus.* In such a case, we at first find a woman full of lasciviousness, almost hysterical in her desire for sex, Eventually, however she becomes absolutely frigid, completely lacking in sexual interest.

Agnus castus patients tend to appear pale, anaemic, fatigued anxious and lacking in courage. They have dilated pupils and sensitivity to light. Their stomachs are easily disordered. If food is the least bit heavy, they will suffer from eating it.

Often there is a sense of inner trembling and coldness — an inner chill. This occurs even though the body itself may feel warm. There is a kind of relaxation of internal organs, and one may see prolapsus and a feeling of weakness in the abdominal area. This is not so much a pressing down sensation, but a weakness. This same weakness can lead also to a Silica-like constipation: the stools come out in pieces, and they sometimes recede.

Sometimes *Agnus castus* is indicated in nursing women whose milk has stopped flowing.

ALUMINA (alum.)

Alumina is a unique remedy often under-appreciated by beginning prescribers. It is characterised by DELAYED ACTION both internally on the mental plane, and externally on the central and peripheral nervous systems. The idea is SLOWNESS of function followed enentually by PARALYSIS. There is a very slow onset. The patient may not realise that anything is wrong for a long time; she may feel a vague "heaviness" in the legs about which she doesn't complain until it has developed into locomotor ataxia.

The most striking aspect of the mental picture is the great SLOWNESS of mind. She is slow to comprehend things, then slow in figuring out how to proceed to accomplish her task, and slow in its execution.

The slowness of mind results in a peculiar kind of confusion which is unique to Alumina. The ideas are very vague, and hazy, like undefined shadows. You may see a patient who has difficulty in swallowing. But when you ask her to describe the trouble, she becomes halting and indecisive. She thinks a long time, tries this word and that, struggling to find the correct word to describe what she is feeling. This difficulty in expressing what is happening is so peculiar to Alumina that it is like a keynote symptom. This is the type of patient whose descriptions are so vague that you may prescribe many remedies before realising that you have never really had a case to work from; once you recognise this peculiar kind of vagueness and confusion, then you will give *Alumina* and witness a good effect.

With time this confusion progresses to another peculiar mental state : when she talks, she thinks that someone else is talking. Or, even more strangely, the patient may say that she cannot hear except through the ears of someone else. This can be tricky, however, because the patient will not volunteer this information. This is the kind of symptom you must elicit by direct questioning. You may suspect Alumina on the basis of other symptoms so you ask about this symptom directly, and the patient says, "Oh yes, now that you mention it."

By this stage of pathology, the patient comes to the conclusion that he or she is going insane. This is not actually a fear of insanity: it is more of an objective conclusion. It is a kind of confirmation of what was previously suspected. Alumina is not a prominent remedy for fear of insanity. In fact, if the patient displays a lot of fear of insanity, one would tend to turn away from *Alumina*.

Finally, the patient falls into a deep sense of despair. She feels, "nobody can help me". "Why am I not getting better"? She feels this over relatively minor ailments, and she goes from doctor to doctor trying to solve the problem; when she sees that no-one can help, then she falls into a despair of recovery. The Arsenicum despair of recovery arises from a tremendous fear of death. In Alumina, however, the despair is very deep, and it is real. She is very sick! The mental plane is confused, she is losing her identity. This can be an early symptomatology of schizophrenia.

It is important to remember that this progression from slowness of mind, to confusion, to loss of identity and despair of recovery, occurs very slowly and eventually the nervous system demonstrates degeneration as well. This is a process seen in broken down constitutions — whether by age or by frequent diseases; it is commonly prescribed in senile patients.

Next we consider the emotional plane. Alumina has a great sense of being hurried inside. Kent stresses this symptom greatly in his Materia Medica, yet Alumina is listed only in ordinary type in the Repertory. What Kent means to say, then, is that this is a sense that the patient cannot do things fast enough; she feels there is such a DELAYED ACTION in functioning that everything happening in the external world seems to move too slowly. This is the basis for the symptoms : "Times passes too slowly". Even though an external observer would see the Alumina patient as being very slow, she feels inside that time is passing too slowly. A half an hour seems to be a whole day.

As the emotional pathology progresses, this sense of being hurried leads to apprehension that she won't be able to finish everything in time. She tries her best, but she is so slow that she cannot actually finish, and this causes her to be apprehensive. At the

Alumina

very extreme of this state, she suffers from a pervasive fear that something bad will happen — an accident, a misfortune.

This process eventually progresses into depression, with suicidal impulses. Alumina has suicidal impulses upon viewing a knife, or seeing blood. Platina, Arsenicum and Mercury are other remedies having a similar symptom, but they mostly have the impulse to kill others. Alumina has the impulse to kill himself or herself.

The Alumina depression can best be described as a "gloominess". There is no light. She complains to the doctor, but in a non-burdensome way. She does not wail and moan and cling to the prescriber. She merely reports her symptoms in a heavy but non-nagging manner. She has the appearance of being RESIGNED to her condition. It has come on over such a long time and so insidiously that she has resigned herself to her condition.

This resignation, coupled with the vagueness and slowness of mind, sometimes gives the patient the appearance of merely "going through the motions". You may observe her a bit and come to the conclusion that she has not really come of her own motivation. She seems to be feeling, "Why did I come here after all?" But then she opens up a bit and begins working with you.

The theme of DELAYED ACTION pervades the physical plane thoroughly. There is a slowing of function at first; this progresses to weakness of muscles, and eventually to a kind of paralysis.

The weakness in Alumina applies peripherally. Just as we see when the patient is struggling so hard to express herself but simply cannot find the right word, she wills herself to function on the plane, but the response is delayed. The characteristic Alumina constipation is the prime example. Here is Kent's description : "Now, so great is the straining to pass a soft stool that you will sometimes hear a patient describe the state as follows : When sitting upon the seat she must wait a long time, though there is fullness and she has gone many days without stool; she has the consciousness that she should pass a stool and is conscious of the fullness in the rectum, yet she will sit a long time and finally will undertake to help herself by pressing down violently with the abdominal muscles, straining vigorously, yet conscious that very little effort is made by the rectum itself. She will continue to strain, covered with copious sweat, hanging on to the seat, if there be any place to hang on to, and will pull and work as if in labour, and at last is able to expel a soft stool, yet with the sensation that more stool remains."

The same thing is seen in the bladder. It takes a long time to get the urine started. In the oesophagus, there is the sensation that food is stuck, that it cannot go down.

The paresis which characterises Alumina is focussed primarily in the legs. The concept of the Alumina loss of identity applies even in this area. The extremities seem to go their own way; they cannot be controlled no matter how hard the patient tries. Thus, we see locomotor ataxia — a clumsy, aimless wobbling of the legs. The same is true of the bladder and rectum — loss of control.

Often a sensation of numbness affects the parts before the onset of the weakness. In particular, there is numbness of the soles of the feet. This typifies the delayed conduction of nerve impulses from the periphery to the brain. As with Cocculus, Alumina displays delayed reflexes upon being pricked with a pin.

There is in Alumina a peculiar kind of vertigo which is frequently observed in neurological cases—vertigo upon closing the eyes. Upon closing the eyes, a patient who is standing will tend to fall over. This again is undoubtedly due to the fact that sensory stimuli from the periphery take too long to provide reliable information to maintain proper balance.

In this way, it is possible to study each system of Alumina and virtually predict what symptoms are seen in the provings. Once the essential themes are understood, the rest falls into place. For example, what kinds of symptoms might be expected in the sexual sphere? There is weakness and loss of control in Alumina, hence the sexual sphere displays diminished desire and, in the male, incomplete or absent erection when there is desire. The genitals are relaxed.

Alumina is known to be one of the main remedies for recurrent colds. How can we explain this? Undoubtedly, it is a relative paralysis of the nerves supplying the mucous membranes. This results in inadequate circulation, or sluggish response of the circulation, along with dryness of the membranes. Since the usual mechanisms whereby the defense mechanism protects against colds have been compromised, the patient becomes susceptible to colds. Basically, this weakness in reactive power is also the basis for pathology in other remedies having colds; Tuberculinum, Sulphur, Graphites, Silica, Mercury.

Some other characteristic physical symptoms : dimness of vision, probably due to weakness of eye muscles. The skin is extremely dry. There is itching without eruption. There are dry crusts on the skin eruptions, dry thick crusts in the nose, and dry granular crusts in the throat. There are catarrhal discharges from all membranes; nasal, urethal, vaginal and easy suppression of discharge which then become recurrent. (There may be one-sided paralysis—usually on the right side.)

Alumina has a definite time aggravation in the morning. She may then gradually improve during the day, or she may remain low all day. However, there is then a marked amelioration in the evening, once the sun has gone down (Medorrhinum, Lycopodium).

Another striking characteristic in Alumina is aggravation from potatoes. There may also be intolerance to other starchy foods, wine, pepper and salt.

The idea of SLOWNESS PROGRESSING INTO PARALYSIS typifies the kind of response which can be expected once Alumina is administered. To be certain of the response it is necessary to wait quite a long time with this remedy. This is especially true when there are organic changes involved. It takes a long time to cure the results of disease, just as it took a long time to develop.

IRRATIONAL THOUGHTS
WHAT MIGHT HAPPEN
LOW SELF CONFIDENCE
likes sugar and fresh air

ARGENTUM NITRICUM (*arg-n.*)

The central idea of the Arg. nit. patient is a person who has a weakness on the mental sphere which is most obvious when a challenge appears. This is a mental weakness accompanied by an emotional state of excitability and nervousness and impulsiveness. His mental faculties are weak while his feelings are overstrong. Such a combination produces a person who is ready to act on any idea which happens to flit through his mind, no matter how ridiculous it may be.

The patient may be sitting on a balcony and suddenly the idea comes to mind; "What if I were to fall?" This idea sticks in his mind and in his imagination he produces the whole scene of falling to the ground and SEEING HIMSELF CRUSHED FULL OF BLOOD etc. Finally, he becomes overwhelmed with this image until he has the actual impulse to jump in order to see what it would be like. He may even make a move toward the edge, but at this moment he comes to his senses—full of fear. He goes inside and he closes the window.

Another example of this combination of weakness and excitability might be a man working on the pavement in the street who finds himself compelled to work in a particular way. If the pavement is laid out in squares, he finds it necessary to work on every other square, or he finds he must step only on the lines between the squares taking very tiny steps.

A further example : A man walking down a street planning to turn a particular corner suddenly becomes obsessed with the thought that the moment he turns that corner a heavy object will fall on him. The thought is so powerful that he continues on past that corner and turns at the next one.

Still another image : A woman crossing the street sees a car passing in front of her at a safe distance. She knows the car cannot hit her and indeed it passes in front of her without incident. Then, as she crosses the street she flashes on a whole scenaris of what MIGHT have happened if she had crossed the street a moment earlier. The vivid image of the car crushing her jolts her back to her senses.

Argentum Nitricum

The Arg. nit. patient becomes temporarily obsessed with such irrational thoughts which possess him for a time and then vanish. A body jerk or sudden movement seems to coincide with the moment the idea leaves.

For example, a man looking from his window sees a child playing in the street. He notices a car which passes the child quite safely. He then starts thinking about what MIGHT have happened had the child been playing in a different part of the street when the car came. He invents a whole horrible scene in his mind and is so carried away by it that he starts down the stairs to the street. As he descends, the idea hits him that he is about to slip and fall. He becomes so overwhelmed by this idea that he is sure it will happen. At this moment, he makes a slightly unusual movement, possibly a jerking motion, and the idea leaves him. He is sane enough to realise that he is constantly tormented by these silly ideas but powerless to stop them.

In Arg. nit. we also find a fear of heights, or a fear of high buildings. The idea behind these two fears is similar : either he will fall from a height, or a building will fall on him as he crosses a street.

For example, a student who has become overtired from too much study sits at his desk and his mind wanders away from his subject. He glances at an electric socket and suddenly wonders : "I wonder what would happen if I put a wire into that socket?" He gets up and finds a wire and starts toward the socket. He comes back to himself with a jerk just as he is about to insert the wire into the socket.

Another patient during an illness becomes absolutely certain that in three hours when the clock strikes a certain hour he will die. He watches the clock in agony. Kent, in the Repertory, under the rubric "Predicts the time of death", lists Aconite, Arg.nit. Agnus castus also should be included. In each of these remedies the idea is quite different. With Aconite, there is a tremendous, overwhelming fear of death which makes him think he is going to die. With Arg. nit. it is a question of a "fixed idea" that he is going to die at a certain hour.

The Arg. nit. person realises that he is weak mentally. He can easily make a fool of himself in public. In a social situation, an overwhelming fear and anxiety may overtake him. He asks himself,

"How shall I ever cope with it? What am I going to do? I shall make such a fool of myself." This anxiety so overwhelms him that he starts to urinate frequently or possibly diarrhoea occurs. This is a state of very low self-confidence. The idea of appearing in public to give a speech seems impossible. The most characteristic aspect of the fears are their "fixed" nature coupled with superstitious paranoia.

To the rubric "Superstitious", which lists Conium and Zincum, should be added Arg.nit., Rhus tox and Stramonium.

The mental weakness manifests throughout the body in ways familiar to us as simple aging. The mental weakness is similar to what we see in senile states. The face appears wrinkled and shrivelled and the patient appears older than his or her actual age. This is not like Calc. carb. which may look old with the furrowing of the face, the fine squares. It is not the same as Lycopodium where the body seems to be aging in the upper half. With Arg. nit. it is more of a shrivelled look (Secale, Ambra grisea).

The Arg.nit. patients emotionally are quite easily over-stimulated. Their emotions are quite strong, even to the point of impulsiveness. They can be very impulsive whether in expressing anger or love. Arg. nit. is the leading remedy for impulsiveness.

It is interesting to note that as the weakened nervous system causes a diminishing of mental function, a corresponding overactivity may occur in the circulatory system. Tremendous palpitations can occur which are felt all over the body, especially while lying on the right side. Flushes of heat can also occur. The Arg. nit. type is aggravated by heat. They like fresh air and cold bathing.

Considering the digestive system, there is a strong desire for sugar and sweets in general, but sugar can disagree, sometimes causing diarrhoea. In addition, there are desires for salt, salty foods and strong cheese. Arg. nit. bloats easily. There is much belching and eructations. The eructations can be continuous and very loud—like cannons. When we have a patient with a strong desire for sugar, a desire for salt who is worse from heat and better from cold, then we must think of Arg. nit. If, in addition, the patient is aggravated by sweets then it is definitely Arg. nit.

The characteristic mental state of Arg. nit. can appear in the sexual sphere as well. He could be emotional and full of feeling but

Argentum Nitricum

as he begins the sexual act he may be overwhelmed with anxiety, causing his penis to relax. This usually occurs because some silly idea has forced itself on him which he cannot let go of. Often the idea is a fearful one, and it renders him incapable of continuing the love act.

Arg. nit has ulcers mostly of the cornea and conjunctiva. Before there is an ulcer there can be a redness in a specific spot.

Stitching, raw pains are also characteristic, not only in the eye, but in the throat as well. It is a "splinter like pain" similar to what we see in Nitric acid and Hepar sulph.

ARSENICUM ALBUM (ars.)

Arsenicum is a classic remedy known in its basic outlines to all homoeopaths. Originally proven by Hahnemann himself, Ars. has been exhaustively described in every Materia Medica since. The classic description in Kent's Materia Medica covers all the essentials in both the acute and chronic states: Anxiety, Restlessness, Aggravated by Cold, Worse 1 - 2 p.m. and 1 - 2 a.m., Thirsty for Sips, Periodicity, Alternations of Symptoms, Ulcerations, Burning PAINS. A mere cataloguing of symptoms can be misleading in actual prescribing. However, unless the image is rounded out by an understanding of the essential dynamic process and stages of development of the remedy, particularly in comparison with other similar remedies.

The essential process underlying the Arsenicum pathology is a deep-seated INSECURITY. From this insecurity springs most of the key manifestations known in Arsenicum. This insecurity is not a mere social dynamic, but more essentially a sense of being vulnerable and defenceless in a seemingly hostile universe. This insecurity dominates the Arsenicum personality even from the earliest stages.

Arising from the insecurity is the Arsenicum DEPENDENCY on other people. Of course, Arsenicum is a prominent remedy listed under the rubric "Desires Company". In reality, the Arsenicum person has more than a mere desire for company—it is an actual need for someone to be present, near him. Arsenicum surrounds himself with people becuase of his insecure sense concerning his health, his unaccountable fear of being alone. The need for company is not necessarily a need for interaction with people, such as in Phosphorus. Arsenicum needs people nearby, more for reassurance and support than anything else.

The Arsenicum person is very POSSESSIVE—possessive about objects, of money, and especially of people. The Arsenicum person does not easily share a relationship with a give and take dynamic. He is much more selfish, a "taker". In a relationship, he will give support to another person, but primarily with the expectation of receiving support in return.

It is in this sense that Arsenicum is a selfish remedy. Automatically, he perceives events in the world from a purely personal standpoint. If something happens to someone else, the Arsenicum person will think first of what it means to him. For example, if a car accident occurs, the Phosphorus patient's heart will automatically go out to the victim, putting himself in the place of the victim. The Arsenicum patient will instantly think to himself,"Oh, Oh! If that can happen to him, it could happen to me." He may not think at all of the other person, but only of the implications to himself.

The possessive quality of Arsenicum extends to physical possessions, as well as people. He is miserly, avaricious. He is conscious of saving money and things, always calculating what the returns to him will be. It can occur that he may be generous with his money or possessions, but he is still giving with the expectation of receiving in return, and he will be upset if the returns do not come back to him. The same possessiveness leads to a compulsive collecting nature. if there is anything that he believes might be of some value even some insignificant little item, he will carefully store it somewhere where he will be able to find it easily later.

Next we come to the well known Arsenicum trait of FASTIDIOUSNESS. Here, it is important first to reiterate that in homoeopathy we do not prescribe on the basis of beneficial traits, but only on pathological qualities. Thus, if someone is neat and orderly as a manifestation of an orderly approach to life, this would not be a limitation in constructing the image of the remedy for that person. The same could be said about the perfectionistic quality, which derives in the same manner as the fastidiousness. On the other hand, we see people who are compulsively fastidious, obsessed by the need for order and cleanliness to the point of expending inordinate energy constantly cleaning and straightening. This is the Arsenicum fastidiousness. It is an obsessive attempt to assuage the anxious insecurity felt inside by creating order and cleanliness in the external world. The fastidiousness in Arsenicum arises out of anxiety and insecurity, whereas in Nux vomica it arises more from an excessive compulsion for work, for overly conscientious attention to details, and to an exaggerated sense of the need for efficiency. The Nat. mur. fastidousness is similar to this, but is more concerned with scheduling of time.

In studying remedies, it is crucially important to have an appreciation of the stages of development of the pathology. Otherwise, if we see a patient at a given stage, we may miss the remedy simply because we are looking for symptoms that are characteristically found at a different stage. Also, an understanding of the stages of a remedy enables us to more readily discern the essence of the remedy and to differentiate it from other similar remedies.

In the early stages of Arsenicum, we see a relative preponderance of physical level symptoms with less emphasis on the mental disturbances. Particular physical complaints, burning pains, chilliness and aggravation from cold, frequent colds periodicity, thirst for sips, and time aggravations of 1 - 2 p.m. or 1 - 2 a.m. may be the primary symptoms to work with. Upon enquiry, one will probably see the fastidiousness, miserliness, and a certain degree of insecurity also. At this stage, particularly if the complaints are more functional and not involving much physical decay, it may be difficult to separate Arsenicum from Nux vomica. One must then search carefully for the psychological tendencies : Arsenicum will tend to be more insecure, needing the support of people, whereas Nux vomica will be more self-reliant and impulsive.

As the illness penetrates deeper, the Arsenicum patient will manifest more anxiety, particularly ANXIETY ABOUT HEALTH, for he is afraid that he will die. At first, this anxiety may be most noticeable upon awakening in the morning, but it gradually occupies his attention throughout the day and night. It is also at this stage that the Fear of Being Alone becomes a prominent factor. He will have a constant need for company, particularly at night. The fears of Arsenicum are raised tremendously while alone.

The Arsenicum anxiety causes great anguish internally, and out of this arises the tremendous restlessness known to this remedy. The restlessness is not a physical process; it is a mental restlessness, an anguished attempt to allay the deep-seated anxiety. He will move from place to place, from chair to chair, from bed to bed. He will go from person to person, constantly seeking reassurance and support.

It is interesting for the homoeopathic prescriber to note the difference between an Arsenicum and Phosphorus patient in rela-

Arsenicum Album

tion to the prescriber. While both have great anxiety about their health, the Phosphorus type will plead for help to the homoeopath, while the Arsenicum type will demand it. The homoeopath is bound to feel the weight with which the Arsenicum patient will cling to him. Once they have reached that stage of development, no patients in our Materia Medica are so clinging and demanding of relief from their anxiety as are Arsenicum and Nitric acid.

It is important to be able to distinguish the peculiar characteristics of the Arsenicum anxiety about health, as there are many other remedies having this characteristic also. The Repertory lists these thoroughly and in relative strengths but it is unable to describe the particular distinguishing qualities which are so important in separating one remedy from another. If one only knows the fact that a particular remedy has the "anxiety about Health" without knowing how to differentiate it from the others, one will find great difficulty in selecting the precise remedy that fits the patient. This cannot be done by a simple process of repertorisation; it requires a minutely detailed knowledge of Materia Medica.

The anxiety about health in Arsenicum is really, deep down inside, a fear of dying. The idea of his own death causes intolerable anguish to the Arsenicum patient. It is not so much the fear of the consequences of a degenerating condition of health, but the fear of the ultimate state of insecurity—death. For this reason the Arsenicum patient will exaggerate many symptoms, blow them out of all proportion. He will come to the conclusion that he has cancer, and will go from doctor to doctor seeking someone who will confirm his fear. Even if all the tests are negative, he will not be consoled; his anguished fear and restlessness will continue to lead him to more and more doctors. He will fear that he has cancer, because that is the symbol of fatal disease in our day and age. It is not really the possibility of cancer, but the prospect of death that causes him such anguish. It is not a fear that he will get cancer some time in the future; he fears that he has it now.

Other remedies have a strong anxiety about health also, but in different ways. Calc. carb. has a strong anxiety about health, but more focussed on the possibility of infectious diesase, or particularly of insanity. Calcarea fears the insanity or the infectious disease itself, not so much the possibility of death. Calcarea can accept death with relative equanimity, but is more likely to be caught in a despair over being incurable and not being able to recover.

Kali. carb. has anxiety that he will get a disease in the future, whereas Arsenicum fears he has cancer now. Kali ars. has a particular anxiety about heart disease, but does not fear death as much as Arsenicum does. The Kali ars. patient will say, "If I must die, it is O.K.", but if you begin talking about his heart he will begin to express anxiety.

Phosphorus feels anxiety about his health, but primarily when the subject is raised to him. Many Phosphorus fears revolve around health, his own or his relatives, but the Phosphorus anxieties are not as obsessive. The Phosphorus patient is suggestible. He hears of someone who has died from a bleeding ulcer, and then he imagines himself to have a bleeding ulcer. He does not hold his anxiety within himself but he will grab the nearest person and animatedly express his concern. He will immediately go to the doctor, who reassures him that he does not have an ulcer; the anxiety then disappears as quickly and easily as it came, to return again on the first provocation. He leaves the doctor's office very relieved, saying to himself, "How silly I am." By contrast Arsenicum, Kali arsenicum and Nitric acid are not so easily pacified. They are inconsolable in their anxieties. The Nitric acid patient, unlike Phosphorus, always has anxiety about his health—an anxiety about any possible ailment, not only cancer, infectious disease, insanity, or heart disease. He may read in a magazine about someone with multiple sclerosis, and he will say to himself, "Oh, Oh! That explains it! That must be what I have". Then, instead of expressing his anxiety, he carries it around inside. Eventually he may very secretively make an appointment with a doctor, but the doctor's assurances fall on deaf ears. He is convinced of what he has and cannot be consoled. Later, he may read another article, and the process begins again. The Nitric acid anxiety about health is not so much the fear of death that we see in Arsenicum, it is more a fear of all the consequences of a long-term degeneration, with the expense, dependency on others, immobility etc.

Lycopodium has a marked anxiety about health. The Lycopodium anxiety can be about any type of illness, like Nitric acid,

Arsenicum Album

but it is an anxiety that springs from a basic cowardice. It is not a fear of death, but a fear of the pain and torture of illness. He has a fear that he won't be able to cope with a serious illness, that he will fall apart and reveal a lack of courage to others.

So it is clear that the simple rubric "Anxiety About Health" is actually full of wide varieties of shades and subtleties which are curcial to the precise choice of a correct remedy. This is true of every rubric, as a matter of fact, in the Repertory.

The same is true of another rubric describing a prominent Arsenicum anxiety—Anxiety for Others. As one would expect from what has already been said, Arsenicum does not have so much of a concern for others per se, but rather a fear of losing someone close to him. Again his anxiety is based on concern for himself. Consequently, he will show little concern over someone who is a stranger to him. It is a fear of loss of someone upon whom he is dependent.

Phosphorus, on the other hand, is so sympathetic and suggestible that he can lose all sense of himself in his concern over someone else, whether a close friend or a stranger. If an Arsenicum person were to meet someone new to the area he would welcome the company but would make conversation merely for the sake of the company; if the person were to mention, say, difficulties in finding a hotel, the Arsenicum patient would courteously express consolation and perhaps make a few suggestions, but his attitude would basically be, "Well, you have your problems but what about the problems I have?" The Phosphorus patient, on the other hand, would become excited and say, "You have no hotel? Oh, my goodness we must do something about that! Here, we'll go right now to the directory and try calling a few!"

Sulpher also has an anxiety about others. In his instance, it is his active imagination which leads to the anxiety. A Sulphur father, for example, might lose sleep worrying about his daughter coming home two hours late from a date. It is not the Arsenicum anxiety over losing his daughter, or the Phosphorus sympathetic anxiety. The Sulphur type will lie awake inventing endless possibilities about what might have happened. He will allow his imagination to blow the whole incident out of proportion to the reality.

Let us return to the stages involved in Arsenicum. The first stage emphasises the physical symptoms, the fastidiousness, and the stinginess. Then we see an increasing emphasis on the insecurities, dependency, anxiety about health, anxiety over losing others, the fear of being alone, and the fear of death. Gradually the fear of death becomes an obsessive, anguishing fear, the central issue of the person's life.

As the illness progresses, we see the emergence of a paranoid, delusionary state. Suspicion dominates the picture. Once the paranoid state develops in a case, we frequently see the fastidiousness disappear. Eventually, the anxiety and fear diminish as a deep state of depression sets in—a despair of recovery, a loss of interest in life, and the suicidal thoughts, suspicion of others and the fear of killing people upon whom he depends. In this stage, the person may even avoid talking to people, becomes obstinate, inward.

It is in this stage of insanity that one may find the most difficulty prescribing Arsenicum without a knowledge of its stages. Many of the usual symptoms of Arsenicum may be missing—anxiety, desire for company, fear of death, restlessness, fastidiousness. It may be difficult to separate Arsenicum from Nux vomica, or other remedies, at this stage. But if the case is taken carefully, the full dynamic process will become clear.

The stages described herein illustrate nicely the progression of pathology steadily into deeper layers of the organism. It begins on the physical level, progressing to a state of anxiety and insecurity, then to fear of death, and finally despair, a loss of interest in life, suicidal disposition and a delusionary state on the mental plane. Consequently, under correct prescribing of Arsenicum in such a case, we can except a reversal of this sequence. As the paranoia and delusions lift and the fears and anxieties return, the homoeopath with a true knowledge of health and disease will recognise progress in the direction toward health.

[Handwritten annotation at top: JOYLESS / REST OF MIND AFTER SUNSET (NORMALLY) / DESTRUCTION OF WILLNESS TO LIVE / + RADIAL]

AURUM METALLICUM (*aur.*)

The main idea essential to Aurum is 'DEPRESSION and LOATHING OF LIFE. Ultimately, this person does not want to live. This idea will be found in practically every Aurum case, whether the patient admits it openly or not.

Aurum patients are closed people. They are not easily able to confess their innermost feelings. In the end, they may freely use the word "depression" but they may be incapable of describing their state more specifically. There are many stages in the development of Aurum pathology, but always they are closed in their relationship with the world.

These are people who feel themselves quite separate from the world. They tend to remain by themselves; they do not have close friends to whom they can turn when they feel depressed or troubled. Usually, they are very proper and correct in their dealings with others—like Kali carbonicum. They are people who are just, honest, fair, and responsible. They would never willingly inflict an injustice on others. They tend to be quite intelligent, hard working and successful. They often attain high positions in society.

Yet, even in the first stages of pathology, these people display a despondency—a dissatisfaction with life in general, especially regarding social and inter-personal relationships. They are closed people who do not express emotions easily. It is as if they are frail on the emotional level; their emotions are not strong enough to be expressed visibly. They are able to accept affection easily from others, but they are not able to return it.

Nevertheless, Aurum patients are characteristically sensitive to any criticism. They are serious minded and they take to heart whatever comments are made about them—similar to Natrum mur. They are too serious to make excuses for another person's harsh remarks—they do not consider the possibility that the person is in a bad mood, under too much stress, not feeling well, etc. In this world view nothing is superficial. Because of their sense of injustice, they may understand the other person's point of view very well but even so they "take it to heart" (an apt phrase for Aurum). They accept the other's to have a different point of view, but then they further conclude that all possibilities of continuing the relationship are lost.

Because of this process, Aurum patients gradually come to the point when they derive no pleasure at all from social or emotional contact. They become joyless. Nothing motivates or excites them.

Aurum patients are people who usually feel they have given a lot of themselves to others, but not in an emotional sense. They often are quite wealthy—financiers, bankers, etc.—and they have given their wealth freely to others, but in return they have been hurt. Consequently they develop resentments which build up inside as a kind of pressure. However, because they are logical and sane people, they try to suppress these negative feelings. They may succeed in this suppression over a period of time, but their emotions then become somewhat unstable. They experience vacillations of moods, changeability.

It is during this stage that Aurum patients are ameliorated in the evening. During the daytime they feel dissatisfied, uncertain, irritable, lacking in self-esteem, feeling unworthy in their occupations etc. In the evening, though there is a return of self-esteem and a relief from the emotional pressures. Even the mind functions better once the sun sets. In this respect, Aurum is similar to Sepia and Medorrhinum. Despite this characteristic, it is also true that in some circumstances Aurum patient; may experience an aggravation of depression in the evening.

As their attempts to suppress negative feelings fail, they break out in tremendous irritability and rage. They may say very damaging things to others. Aurum patients at this stage of pathology may seem cruel and unfeeling to others, especially in their manner of speaking. They do not actually curse—they are too proper for that—but they may say very harsh and violent things to people around them.

In an attempt to control the poisonous process which seems to be overtaking the emotional level, Aurum patients turn more and more to mental activity. They are very industrious and hard-working, but to a pathological degree. Work becomes an outlet to avoid the discomfort of an emotional life which has become increasingly isolated and undernourished.

Aurum Foliatum

They eventually feel as if they have completely failed in life, that they are only taking others into believing they are capable, worthwhile individuals. They feel that they do not deserve their status, wealth and responsibilities. They begin to feel that they have no right to live, and that they are literally incapable of maintaining their occupations or relationships. They put the blame for everything on themselves. It is during this stage that Aurum patients become exquisitely sensitive to even chance remarks by others. For the most trivial of reasons, they may jump out of a high window and everyone is surprised. There did not seem to be any big problems and things seemed to be functioning smoothly. But no-one realised the depth of suffering these individuals reach inside.

Finally, even the work strategy fails, and they become suddenly overwhelmed by depression, sadness, and grief. At this point, all is completely without hope. Everything becomes darker and darker, until there seems to be not one ray of light. To these Aurum patients, it is as if the sun has been completely snuffed out and there is no longer any point in continuing to live.

By this stage, all the destruction which used to be turned outward in their resentment, irritability and rage, now turns inward. Their thoughts turn constantly to suicide. They feel only a gloom and sadness; life is no longer worthwhile in any sense. They reach the deepest states of depression of which human beings are capable.

In a recent newspaper article, there was a story about a man who shot his wife, his two children, and himself, because he THOUGHT he was going to lose his job. This was very likely an Aurum case. It is interesting that Aurum patients value gold (money) a lot. Their material positions are very important to them. This is one of the reasons why they are so industrious. They may work hours of overtime, partly to ensure their financial security, but also to help allay the feeling that they do not deserve their position.

Classically, the image of Aurum suicidal thinking has been that they have the impulse to jump from a high place. In all their misery and gloom, when they look over high edge, the idea overtakes them. "Now, one jump and there will be relief". They are overtaken by a kind of cloud, a sweet feeling that if they jump everything will be finished. Nowadays, however, there is another kind of impulse. Especially during a fit of rage or despondency, they may get into a car and recklessly push the accelerator to the floor in the hope of losing control. Or there may be an impulse to swerve the car into a wall or an embankment.

The Aurum state represents a true living death, a complete destruction of the mind and the will to live, illness beginning on the emotional plane.

It is interesting that Aurum patients, being very proper and moralistic, may take another course in their pathology, leading to religious behaviour. Instead of becoming truly suicidal, they tend to pray constantly for salvation. This praying is often accompanied by weeping, and this seems to relieve them. The tremendous gloom and sadness they feel is relieved by praying and weeping hour upon hour.

I remember a schoolmate of mine in India who had painful swelling of the testes. He was a nice person and showed no real signs to casual observation of difficulty on the emotional plane. He saw several of the homoeopathic professors who gave him Clematis, Rhododendron, and other remedies, all with no effect. The pain was very severe, so he finally consulted me. At the end of the interview he said, "You know, I am a Christian and I like it, but every night before I go to sleep I feel compelled to pray for one or two hours. I cannot do otherwise". Upon enquiry, it turned out that he was in actuality quite depressed, but never had thoughts of suicide. Aurum was given, and after an aggravation for a few hours, it completely relieved him within three days.

Sometimes Aurum is indicated in children, but they will not show the depression. They will, however, tend to be serious, overly responsible, changeable in moods, irritable with fits of anger, and moaning and lamenting.

It is interesting also that there is a correspondence between the emotional level and heart disease. If, for example, an Aurum patient finds a solution to his problems by other means—divorce and a new love, or some other method—then we may see the appearance of cardiac disorders. There may also be heart disease arising out of suppression of rheumatoid diseases; Aurum is a prominent remedy to consider in easy suppressions affecting the heart.

Whenever there is even a trivial heart ailment, Aurum patients develop a fear of heart disease. Whatever anxiety about health which exists in Aurum patients is focussed on the heart. This is not a fear of death. Aurum patients, when asked about whether they fear death, usually answer, "No, not at all. I welcom death. This is no life to live". Yet, they do have a fear of heart disease, which represents the plane of emotional vulnerability.

Aurum sometimes is prescribed for very severe rhinitis with offensive odour. The odour is so offensive that even others can smell it.

The syphilitic element is evident in Aurum. They have the typical deep bone pains of the syphilitic miasm.

Also Aurum covers all pains, of whatever origin, which drive the patient to want to commit suicide. The pains become so severe that death seems the only possible relief. I remember a case of neuralgia of one of the nasal branches of the trigeminal nerve. It was an incredible pain that drove the patient completely mad and she wanted to die. It was, quickly relieved by Aurum 10 M. I recall another case of severely painful mastoditis which was recurrent for years; this was also promptly cured by Aurum.

Aurum is a remedy which is capable of reaching into the deepest regions of the human organism when properly indicated and it is sometimes astounding to see the changes it can produce. Patients with deep-seated depressions develop a true elation about life; because of the previous darkness they truly appreciate the new found light they feel inside.

[Handwritten annotations at top: DELAYED DEVELOPMENT / FEAR OF STRANGERS / VACANT MIND – INABILITY TO HANDLE COMPLICATION / CHILDISH BEHAVIOUR]

BARYTA CARBONICA (bar-c.)

Baryta carb. is a remedy which can be prescribed at all stages of life—childhood, adulthood, old age—but it is most commonly indicated in children. This remedy brings aid to scrofulous children, especially if they are backward physically, are dwarfish, do not grow and develop.

The dwarfishness is seen not only on the physical level but on the emotional and mental levels as well.

By dwarfishness we do not mean that Baryta carb. is routinely prescribed for people who are short in stature, or for actual dwarfs. It is not indicated in people with quick intelligence and strong vitality. Baryta carb. dwarfishness on the physical plane refers more specifically to conditions in which specific organs have not fully developed, especially the genitalia. The testes and penis may be very small and relaxed. Or the uterus may remain child sized even into adulthood. Delayed development in general is a strong element in Baryta carb.

The appearance of Baryta carb. children is quite distinct. They are not fat, but they may have enlarged bellies with an otherwise marasmic appearance—like Calcarea carb. The skin is not fresh, as it is in most children; it appears older, as if it is about to become wrinkled. The glands may be swollen, and especially the tonsils may swell to such an extent that it interferes with the child's appetite. Because of this adenoidal and tonsillar swelling, the child may breathe through his mouth, which adds to the generally "stupid" look on his face. Baryta carb. children have a very serious look on their faces. There is an unintelligent seriousness to their mind. They lack brilliance, so they appear as if they are always trying to figure out what is happening. It is as if the mind is completely vacant.

These children are very shy. In the interview, a Baryta carb. girl will hide behind the chair and cling to her mother, peering out at you with that dull, serious look. You cannot coax her to come out. If you go over and take her by the hand, however, she will not resist. Other remedies—like Natrum mur, Tarentula, Arnica, or Hepar children—will kick up a fuss if you make a move toward them; they know how they feel and they will not allow you to touch them. The Baryta carb. child, however, will allow you to bring her to you.

She is docile. She may stare at you, wondering "What does this man want of me?" But she has no will of her own. She will try to do whatever you wish. It is a shyness that comes from a lack of comprehension and an instinct to remain in familiar circumstances and with familiar people who can protect her. It should be pointed out, also, that this shyness may persist until the age of 8 or 10 years. It is natural for children 3 or 4 years to be shy, but in Baryta carb. it persists to a much older age and exactly the same childishness. This is why Bartya carb. is listed in the Repertory as having a fear of strangers and aversion to company.

Baryta carb. children are slow to learn—to walk, and especially to talk. They may not learn to talk until the age of 3 or 4 years. You stand them on their feet, to teach them to walk, but they simply do not seem to comprehend that they are supposed to put one foot in front of the other. In a normal school, these children fall behind quickly; it is common for them to hold back a year every three years or so until they receive Baryta carb.

In Greek, there is a word, MICRONOUS, which means "small mind" or "simplemindedness". This is an accurate description of the Baryta carb. intellect. Their minds seem completely incapable of handling complexities—any problem involving more than 4 or 5 factors, for example. They tend to think in a rote fashion. Structure and routine are best for them.

A father may ask his Baryta carb. son to study a passage in the history book for class the next day. He willingly sits there for a long time applying himself to the passage and by the end of the time he can recite it from memory. However, he has not really comprehended its meaning. The next day, the teacher asks him to describe that passage, and he simply cannot respond. Partly he is overcome by shyness, but mostly he has forgotten the passage completely. The Baryta carb. mind is vacant; it cannot comprehend easily, cannot retain things.

These children realise that they don't understand all that happens in the world around them. This is why they tend to stay by themselves, in familiar and safe surroundings. They will not play with other children. They will not make new friends. This also is the reason why they have anxiety about others; they are fearful of losing their protectors, their familiar relations.

Of course, one might think of Baryta carb. for mongoloid children. One must be careful, however, to distinguish conditions which are pathological and actual defects. In mongoloids, there is a specific defect; there is only a certain amount of intelligence available at birth. The intelligence which is lacking from the outset cannot be brought to normal. However, mongoloid children sometimes have other problems, susceptibilities to colds, etc. which can be helped by various remedies such as Calc. carb., Tuberculinum, Pulsatilla, and others.

This description of Baryta carb. carried on into adulthood as well, but usually these people have learned to compensate for their lack of intelligence. In social gatherings, they remain silent while everyone else speaks. Generally, they shun society and stick close to their own family.

It is in adulthood, however, that the CHILDISH behaviour becomes most evident. They say things that seem to have no relation to the topic being discussed—silly things, ridiculous things. For example, people are discussing popular music, and someone remarks that Elvis Presley is a great performer. Then the Baryta carb. man says, "Yes, he's O.K. but he cannot compare to Maria Callas!" This is the kind of silly, out-of-context remark that Baryta carb. patients make. They seem to lack perspective altogether, so their minds make only the simplest of connections, which seem ridiculous and childish to other people.

Let us take another example, Baryta carb. patients can perform their routine daily functions quite adequately, but they cannot cope with extra complications. Suppose a man tells his wife that ten people are coming to dinner. She is perfectly capable of cooking for just herself and her husband, but ten people? She can't cope with the complexity of which utensils to use, how to time things so that all the food is ready at the same time, etc. She doesn't know where to begin or where to end. But instead of saying this straight out, she says to her husband,"But I do not have the right shoes to wear!"

It is this inability to handle complexity that leads to the IRRESOULTION which is so characteristic of Baryta carb. Suppose a man and wife are looking for a new house, and one is offered

Baryta Carbonica

at a bargain. It is a perfect sized house, located in a very nice area, and the price is the only one quarter of the usual market value for such houses. The husband asks, "What do you think?" The wife realises that this is the moment for a decision: they have saved their money, but now she is afraid of the magnitude of th decision. So she says "Yes, but that mountain nearby is so big; it may cut off the air! And there is dirt on the porch". She has no ability to put things in their correct perspective, so she cannot come to a decision. It is like asking a child to make the decision on buying a house. Whenever irresolution is the major expression on the mental level, Bartya carb. is one of the main remedies to consider.

Because the mind is so simple in Bartya carb. they do not have the burden of over-intellectualisation. Often they can be quite receptive and accurate in an intuitive way. Upon meeting someone, they will immediately intuit whether that person is good or bad, and they will often be right. Even so, their judgement will be quite complex. They are not really capable of very subtle or refined impressions.

Bartya carb. is a remedy which can be indicated in old arteriosclerotic people whose minds have deteriorated in a specific way. These are old people who play with dolls, or tie ribbons in their hair—childish behaviour. In such people, Bartya carb. may well bring them back to their normal selves for another two or three years until the inevitable decline overtakes them.

Bartya carb. and Baryta mur. are often indicated in mononucleosis, when the glands have become swollen and very hard.

Generally, Bartya carb. patient are chilly. They often have an aversion to sweets. Baryta carb. is one of only three remedies which have an aversion to fruits, and especially to plums.

A peculiar symptom which might lead you to Baryta carb. is the sensation that they are inhaling smoke when in fact the air is clean.

Handwritten annotations at top:
- FEAR OF BEING ALONE DURING THE PAIN
- BACK MASSAGE RELIEVES PAIN & ANXIETY
- THIRST FOR COLD DRINKS, THEN VOMITING WHEN THEY BECOME WARM
- PERIODIC PAROXYSM

BISMUTHUM SUBNITRICUM (bism.)

Bismuth is a very distinct remedy which is needed in a specific situation in which no other remedy can replace it. Its characteristics are such that it will very easily be confused with Phosphorus. Bismuth is indicated in certain specific cases in which there is very severe, violent pain in the stomach. The patient complains of a very severe cramping pain, as if something is grasping the stomach. The pain is so severe that the patient is in a constant turmoil, writhing about in great distress. The arms, the legs, the whole body—all are in constant motion. The pain is so great that the patient is in great fear. He or she keeps saying "Am I going to be well?
Am I going to get better? Please hold me! Do not leave me alone." These patients because of the violence of the pain, have a great fear of being left alone. They need somebody to be with them at all times—sometimes just to hold their hands. This fear of being alone during the pain is very characteristic for a Bismuth.

Another keynote of Phosphorus which these people have is a great thirst—especially for cold water and in large quantities. Then, once they drink the water, they may stick a finger into the throat in order to immediatly vomit it up. Alternatively, if they do not artificially induce vomiting, the water will be vomited up only once it has become warm in the stomach. This symptom in particular may make you think of Phosphorus—especially when combined with the tremendous anxiety about health, the need for reassurance and the desire for company during the pain.

Another striking characteristic is that the pain is ameliorated by rubbing or massaging the back. Massagaing the region of the solar plexus itself cannot be tolerated, but rubbing the opposite region of the back ameliorates. This may relieve not only the pain itself, but also the tremendous anxiety and writhing about.

The pain itself is centred in the solar plexus. At first, it may feel like a heartburn, but soon it becomes a severe cramping gastralgia, as if something were going to break inside. The pain becomes so intolerable that you are likely to decide immediately upon hospitalisation, and the pain continues unabated for days.

The pain in Bismuth lasts continuously for days at a time, but the paroxysms have an approximate periodicity to them. The periodicity may be every 15, 30 or 45 days; but once the paroxysm begins, its violence and characteristic anxiety, accompanied by great thirst for cold drinks which are vomited, is unmistakeable.

During the paroxysm of pain, of course, no food can be tolerated whatsoever. It is strange, however, that once the pain abates, these patients can eat and digest virtually anything—even stones.

During the paroxysm of pain, the body and head may feel as if there is a fever. Eventually the extremities become cold, but the torso and head remain warm to the touch, even though there is no actual fever.

Bismuth is a wonderful remedy to remember for this specific situation. You may be called to the patient's home and everyone is in a panic beacause of the violence of the symptoms. Obviously, no ordinary antispasmodics would be capable of dealing with such pains, and an allopathic prescriber would be forced to consider either very powerful drugs or surgery. The symptoms themselves cannot fail to bring to your mind Phosphorus, but Phosphorus will not touch such a case. It is too violent, too extreme.

Also, as a general rule, Bismuth can be kept in mind for even milder gastralgias in seemingly Phosphorus-type patients but in whom Phosphorus has failed to provide any benefit. After trying Phosphorus and waiting sufficiently long for a response, Bismuth could be considered as a further possibility, especially when there is history of periodicity to the paroxysms.

AGGRAVATION FROM BODY MOTION
IRRITABILITY
RESIGNATION

AMELIORATION FROM PRESSURE

BRYONIA (bry.)

The descriptions which characterise Bryonia are LONELINESS and INSECURITY. Bryonia patients are witdrawn into themselves, purposely isolated from social contact. Always in the background is a deep feeling of insecurity, a sense of vulnerability and weakness. It is this that leads them to seek isolation. They do not want to be intruded upon, and they are quite content to live alone.

Bryonia patients are very sensitive to any intrusions; they are quick to feel irritability, anger and resentment. Inside, they feel great unhappiness and despondency. Especially during acute ailments, they feel dull in the mind and despondency on the emotional level. They do not want to show this however. They just want to be left alone.

The most well-known major keynote of Bryonia, of course, is AGGRAVATION FROM ANY MOTION, applies on all three levels. The mind is dull; it cannot take any exertion at all, even that of the simplest conversation. In acute conditions, this dullness of mind is a very prominent characteristic which must be emphasised. Emotionally, any imposition—even consolation or well-meaning attempt to help—is met with immediate irritation and resentment. And of course the physical body suffers from every motion. The Bryonia patient wants to lie perfectly still in a dark room, being left completely alone. Even turning on a light will set up a reaction because even the very slight movement of the iris will cause an aggravation; the Bryonia patient cannot even take that!

A Bryonia man who is suffering from the flu will isolate himself, turn out the light, and lie in bed without the slightest movement. If his wife quietly slip into the room and asks if he wants some warm tea, he will feel irritated by even this question, in spite of its loving intent. He will automatically and emphatically say "No!" If she persists and brings the tea anyway, he may drink it and feel ameliorated, because Bryonia is very thristy. In spite of this thirst, however, his initial response will usually be negative because he doesn't want to be bothered by anything.

Bryonia

The irritability of Bryonia patients is such that they seem to hold other people responsible for their suffering. They are aggressive in a manner which makes others feel uneasy.

In spite of the outward aggressiveness, Bryonia patients feel very insecure inside—especially about their financial well-being. When they feel ill, the first thing they want to do is go home, where they feel secure from any stress. In a delirium, they talk mostly of business because they fear for their financial security. This is most dramatically demonstrated by the fact that Bryonia is the most prominent remedy listed under Fear of Poverty.

Bryonia patients, then are quite materialistically-minded (although not as much as Arsenicum). Even idealistic people will have a deep sense of insecurity regarding their financial future. In actual fact, they may be quite secure financially, but they have an irritational fear that they are headed toward bankruptcy. Of course, this refers to a pathological fear of poverty, not one which is based in actual reality.

It seems to me that this insecurity arises out of the lack of social contact in Bryonia patients. They do not allow themselves the sense of security that can be derived from family, friends, community etc. Bryonia patients are responsible people; they usually take the greatest share of responsibility for their families, for instance, but then they wonder who will take care of THEM in case of financial disaster. They feel unsupported and insecure. The suffering of Bryonia patients, of course, is very great—whether in acute ailments, migraine headaches, or chronic arthritic pains. Every movement aggravates them greatly. This suffering can lead to a fear that they are going to die, but more commonly they fall into a despondent state. They seem to give up and simply accept the apparent inevitability that they are going to die. This is a despair of recovery, but it is not full of the agony that is found in Arsenicum or Calc. carb It is a resignation to what seems to be inevitable.

On the physical level, of course, there are many symptoms for which Bryonia is quite famous. The aggravation from motion is the most prominent. You must remember, however, that if the pains become too severe in Bryonia, they may become very restless. The suffering becomes so intense that they feel compelled to do something, and then they start moving about. In this situation, Bryonia can be mistaken for Rhus tox or Arsenicum. However, despite the restlessness, the Bryonia pains are still not ameliorated by motion.

Another keynote of Bryonia is amelioration from pressure. They want to hold the painful part, to tie up the head, or to lie on the painful side. This amelioration from pressure, coupled with aggravation from motion, explains why Bryonia is considered virtually a specific remedy in appendicitis. Physicians everywhere know the classic clinical sign by which appendicitis is diagnosed—rebound tenderness. Slowly and gently pressure is applied over the appendix, but no pain is felt until the pressure is let up with a snap—amelioration from pressure but aggravation from motion. Of course, appendicitis can present itself in other ways, but most commonly fits these two main keynotes of Bryonia. I recall one appendicitis case that was seen by one of the doctors in our centre. It was so obvious that he felt compelled to send the boy to the hospital. I told him to give a dose of Bryonia first, and by the time he was examined at the hospital, the doctor could find no evidence for appendicitis.

Generally Bryonia is a left-sided remedy, particularly in migraine headache. Migraines are usually one-sided at first, and Bryonia most often fits those on the left side which are better from pressure and the application of a cold wet towel. These headaches are congestive in nature, sometimes with flushing and may eventually involve the whole head.

Another characteristic symptom on the physical level is the great dryness of the mucous membranes. This dryness is a general symptom; it even applies to the emotional level. Bryonia patients are emotionally dry; there is not much happening on the emotional plane. Naturally, dryness of the mucous membranes lead to great thirst—frequently, and for large quantities. It does not matter in Bryonia whether the water is warm or cold. Even if the desire is for cold water, it will never be as greatly stressed as in Phosphorus (again emphasising the importance of underlining in a written case). Whenever there is stomach trouble (gastritis, duodenal ulcer, etc.) however, Bryonia wants warm drinks, which ameliorate.

It must be remembered, however, that Bryonia is also one of the main remedies for dryness with thirstlessness, along with Belladonna, Nux moschata, and Natrum mur.

Bryonia often has an afternoon time aggravation—around 3 or 4 or even 7 p.m. Most characteristic, though is a 9 p.m. aggravation lasting until sleep. This can be a strong confirmatory symptom for Bryonia whenever it is present, just as 9 a.m. aggravation can suggest Chamomilla.

There are not many strong symptoms in Bryonia regarding desires and aversions. Many times there may be a desire for oysters, but that is all. As mentioned, warm drinks ameliorate the stomach troubles.

Bryonia patients suffer from vertigo, especially on turning the head to look backward. Turning in bed also creates vertigo, as one might expect. Usually Bryonia patients want to lie on the left side and are aggravated by lying on the right side.

Bryonia is a remedy which is slow to develop in its pathology and slow in its action once given. In chronic Bryonia cases, you will see a long history of gradual development—say, over a period of five years. In arthritis, first one joint will be mildly affected, then another. By contrast, arthritic pains in Formica rupha erupt dramatically in several joints at once. Over the year, though, the inflammations increase in number and intensity until the patient becomes a total wreck—and even full of anxiety and restlessness because of the intensity of the pains. At this point Bryonia can be confused with Rhus tox because the rheumatic pains are ameliorated by warmth (congestive pains in Bryonia are ameliorated by cold).

Acute Bryonia cases develop over a period of days. Perhaps there is an exposure to cold, but few symptoms occur for the first few days. A fever may appear by the third day or so, and then a full-blown illness is apparent by the fourth day. This same progress is true of Gelsenium. By contrast, Belladonna or Aconite erupt like volcanoes in their symptomatology.

Once you have seen an acute Bryonia case you are not likely to forget it. I remember the first acute case I ever treated—a man with bronchitis. I visited him in his home, where he lived with another single man. As I entered his room, he was sitting on the bed facing the wall, his back turned to me. I asked "How are you? How do you feel?" He would not answer me, nor would he turn to face me. Throughout the entire interview I was unable to get him to turn around. His fever was very high and he had such a painful cough that he had to hold his chest and let out weak little coughs. When I asked what he ate, his friend replied that he only took water. Obviously, this was a perfect Bryonia case, and he rapidly recovered.

DISCONTENTMENT
EFFORT TO OVERCOME PROLONGED STRESS
ANXIETY ABOUT FUTURE → HEALTH

CALCAREA CARBONICA (*calc.*)

Calcarea carbonia is a very broad remedy with many ramifications. Perhaps the best way to describe it is to take each of the three levels separately.

The fundamental disturbance of calcium metabolism which Calc. carb. epitomises seems to manifest in two different body types. Most Calc. carb. cases, of course, are the *fair, fat, flabby* types so well described in the literature. These people gain weight easily and have difficulty losing it even when consuming very few calories. This is so characteristic of Calc. carb. that it is almost always present. There is another type of appearance which can occasionally be seen; a *lean, thin, person with a lean face covered by fine wrinkles*. The fine wrinkles are arranged in *horizontal and vertical lines* producing *small squares;* the overall appearance is of a person who has *suffered a great deal*. This lean type of Calc. carb. patient undergoes all the typical stages of Calcarea pathology, even though his or her appearance does not resemble the classic stereotype.

It is interesting that a large percentage of infants and children seem to need Calc. carb. Although *it should never be prescribed routinely.* to infants or children, it is neverthelss true that it is probably the most commonly prescribed remedy in the age group. To me, this fact suggests that one of the most fundamental disturbances in the human organism is that which affects calcium metabolism.

It is for this reason that whenever you encounter a patient *60 or 70 years of age* who clearly needs Calc. carb., you can be assured that the patient has *a basically strong constitution*. Typically, these elderly Calc. carb. patients have lived active lives with very few health problems. Finally perhaps due to over-exertion or excessive life stresses, they show some pathology. In such cases, the prognosis is quite good. *Anyone who can maintain into old age the same remedy image which is characteristic of childhood can be said to have a basically sound constitution.*

Calc. carb. childern present a fairly typical picture. They are generally somewhat plump, soft, and flabby. Their compleions tend to be rather waxy and pale. They do not have much stamina, so they *generally avoid physical activities*. By nature they are rather *reserved, withdrawn and self-reliant*. They would rather sit and watch than, actively join the games of other children.

Calc. carb. children definitely display a tendency to *profuse perspiration*. This may arise after even slight exertion, but most characteristically it comes on within the *first ten minutes or so of sleep*. The perspiration is most *prominent* in the (cervical region) than in the *head and face*, and finally the upper torso. In children, the lower torso is almost never affected, although adult Calc. carb. patients may perspire there as well. In adults, *there is a clammy sweat of the palms and feet*. Also adults are likely to sweat even in a cold environment; there is some unusual reaction in the body which causes them to *perspire in the cold*.

Calc. carb. children usually have a history of frequent colds during the winter and a strong tendency toward glandular swellings. *Calc. carb. are usually constipated, but they do not notice it themselves, nor do they suffer from it*. It is the mother who notices that the child has gone 3 or 4 days without a bowel movement, and then she becomes concerned. This is characteristic for Calc. carb. children and they generally *feel better when they are constipated*. It is *when the diarrhoea comes on that they begin to whine and complain and feel discontented*.

The situation is reversed in adulthood. The condition of the bowels is frequently a major focus of attention in *adult* Calc. carb. patients. Here, the opposite situation holds true; *diarrhoea relieves* and constipation aggravates the patient. It is interesting how frequently such reversals occur in different stages of many remedies in homoeopathy.

The typical aggravation from *cold wet weather* seen in adults *is not exhibited in Calc. carb. children*. Sometimes one might be misled into believing they are actually warm-blooded people because of the perspiration. They perspire from the slightest exertion. Also, the perspiration during early sleep may cause them to throw covers of the upper half of the body.

Calc. carb. children exhibit a definite desire for *soft-boiled eggs and for sugar*.

Calc. carb. children usually are good students once they get into

Calcarea Carbonica

school. *They are intelligent, but their comprehension may be a bit slow.* It takes them a bit longer to understand the material being presented, and for this reason they *often feel hurried in their work. They are capable of hard work*, however, and they may spend hours completing their homework.

If Calc. carb. pathology reaches into the emotional plane during childhood, *you may see a lot of whining and moaning, a discontentment.* You ask the child what he wants, and he *cannot tell you.* It is a state of complaining and dissatisfaction.

Also, between the ages of about six and twelve Calc. carb. children commonly develop *an intense curiosity about supernatural things*, the unknown, the beyond. They seriously ask such questions as, "What is God? What does God intend to do with us? Who are the angels? How do angels behave? Why do people die? What happens to us after death?" These questions, of course, depend on the type of background of the child, and they are natural in many children. In Calc. carb. children, however, this curiosity can be carried to a pathological extreme. Such a child may say she is actually waiting for an angel to come and take her to paradise.

I cannot exactly explain this predilection in Calc. carb. children. It seems to arise out of the observation of the world around them. They see suffering and injustices; perhaps there is some conflict between the parents. Then someone mentions God and this concept seems to penetrate readily into their minds. God, angels, and supernatural influences seem to explain the world to them. They keep on thinking about these things, asking questions and imagining various fancies.

In adulthood, this predilection expresses itself as a *fear of insanity.* In Calc. carb. the *fear of insanity is a fear of losing control, a fear of the unknown.* These people have learned to resort to the mind a great deal, to rely upon it to overcome difficulties. Consequently, when they finally collapse under too much stress and overexertion, the major fear is that of losing the mind, their primary means of maintaining control.

In Calc. carb. pathology comes on under the *demands of stress and a prolonged effort to overcome it.* They are able people, generally healthy under ordinary circumstances. However, prolonged stress and overexertion finally leads to a breakdown, first on the physical level, and later on the emotional and mental levels. *Overexertion—either physical or mental,—is the greatest enemy of Calc. carb. patients.*

Pathology on the physical level in the adult Calc. carb. patient primarily affects the musculo-skeletal system. Rheumatism and arthritis are the main manifestations on the physical level. In the adult, there is definitely an aggravation from cold, wet weather, and an amelioration from warmth. The first region affected in Calc. carb. patients is the *lumbar region*. The trouble starts there and then *spreads to the cervical region and out to the extremities*. Whenever you see a patient who is slightly obese, affected by cold wet weather, and his main complaints centre around arthritis and rheumatism, there is already a strong possibility of Calc.carb.

Calc. carb. patients have cold extremities. They *wear socks to bed at night*. However, they end up taking the socks off later in the night because the feet begin to burn.

Simultaneously with the emotional plane, the mental level begins to break down as well. They tend *to focus on little things,* to obsess about irrelevant details. They make *silly little jokes,* or *they keep talking about insignificant things which are unimportant to anyone else.*

At this point, the previous anxiety about the future gives way to *anxiety about health*. There is *fear of infectious diseases,* of tuberculosis, of heart disease, of cancer etc. Nowadays, Calc. carb. patients are particularly susceptible to fears of cancer and heart disease. Naturally, there is a strong fear of death.

Eventually, this fear-ridden state leads of a *hysterical* state. They seem *to lose their powers of comprehension and concentration*. They *don't know what they want,* and they become very agitated. *They pace up and down.* They have impulses to smash things, to jump out of the window, to shout and scream. All this is without provocation, or very little provocation. They are in a *state of turmoil,* and they *just want to shout or do something desperate.*

At this point, these patients truly are on the verge of insanity. If they do progress into true schizophrenia or other psychosis, however, another remedy will most likely be needed. In my experience, Calc. carb. is not indicated in an actually psychotic patient.

Calcarea Carbonica

A characteristic symptom which appears in Calc. carb. as the mental plane breaks down is the *fear that others will observe their confusion*. They are aware of the dullness of mind, the inability to sustain their concentration, and the resulting confusion. They live in dread that this confusion will be discovered by others. This, however, is a symptom, that Calc. carb. patients will never voluntarily divulge. You must ask this question directly in order to confirm it. Usually they will answer you with an emphatic "Yes!" and a tremendous expression of relief. They feel so grateful that someone else understands.

During the development of mental and emotional pathology, you will very likely see a disappearance of many physical symptoms. First to go, of course, is the perspiration. These deeply suffering people may not be as affected by cold wet weather. They may still feel the cold, but not nearly so emphatically as previously. The desire for eggs and sweets may disappear altogether.

At this stage, it can be easy to confuse Calc. carb. with Phosphorus. If the patient retains the typical thirst for cold drinks, the desire for ice cream, and the desire for salt, the decision can be quite difficult. The anxiety about health, fear of death, and suggestible fears of cancer and heart disease can suggest Phosphorus as well as Calc. carb. Calc. carb. can have fear of thunderstorms and fear of the dark. Calc. carb. often has heart palpitations which resemble Phosphorus.

There are a few points which can differentiate Calc. carb. from Phosphorus, however. *Calc. carb. does not need company nearly as much as Phosphorus.* Calc. carb. *tends to sleep on the left side*, whereas Phosphorus prefers to sleep on the right. *Calc. carb. prefers hot food*, whereas Phosphorus wants cold food. Both can be very thirsty for cold water, but this is much more strongly emphasised in Phosphorus; such thirst in Calc. carb. would be underlined once, or at the very most twice, whereas it would be underlined two or three times in Phosphorus. Finally, the physical appearance is quite different. Phosphorus is tall, thin, and delicate. Calc. carb. usually is obese and flabby; even the lean Calc. carb. patient is full of wrinkles and not so delicate in appearance.

Handwritten notes at top:
DIFFICULTY IN CONCENTRATION
DISCONTENT
MIND & MUSCLES BECOME FLABBY

CALCAREA PHOSPHORICA (calc-p.)

Calc. phos. is a remedy which probably is not adequately appreciated. It is very deep-acting remedy with a wide spectrum of symptomatology, but it is easy to mistake for other remedies more classically know as "polychrests". I kown in my own practice that I have frequently given Calc. carb., Phosphorus, Phosphoric acid, and even Chamomilla when I should have given Calc. phos. Gradually, however, I have learned to discern a few points which distinguish it from other remedies. In this chapter I shall try to highlight these characteristics, along with the most striking points of its general symptomatology.

DISCONTENT is the main theme around which the image of Calc. phos. develops. Calc. phos. patients do not know what they want. They know something has gone wrong with their system, but they do not know precisely what it is or what to do about it. A sluggishness has affected the whole organism, and this brings about a deep discontent, a deep dissatisfaction.

In Calc. phos., there is usually a specific moment in time when the person's energy suddenly decreased. Perhaps there was an acute ailment, a shock of some sort, penicillin injections, etc. Whatever the cause, there followed a quite rapid decline of energy—not overnight perhaps, but over a brief period of time. Then, from that moment, the patient noticed a sluggishness of mind, an emotional indifference, and a lack of physical stamina. This state of lowered vitality usually affects all three levels simultaneously in Calc. phos., and it is this which leads to the pervasive discontent.

In Calc. phos., the fundamental weakness is seen most dramatically on the mental plane. It is as if the mind has become flabby in the same way that muscles become flabby. Here the Calc. carb. element is quite evident. The mind seems to slow down to about one-third its normal speed. This is not a perversion of mental function or a confusion. The mental processes function properly, but only at a much slower rate and requiring much more effort than previously. A Calc. phos. patient can do mathematics, for

Calcarea Phosphorica

instance, but a problem that used to take a half-hour prior to the onset of pathology now takes an hour and a half.

Then, because of the effort involved, he begins to make mistakes—to miswrite letters or to misplace words. It becomes difficult to concentrate the mind. The patient becomes forgetful, she goes into another room to get something, only to forget what it was once she gets there.

A normal healthy person is capable of generating thoughts, a flow of ideas, some degree of reflection. The Calc. phos. patient loses this capacity. If there is time, and no distractions, he can complete the task at hand, but only slowly and with effort. However, the interesting thing is that Calc. phos. patients can be STIMULATED to work to their previous capacity if the task is sufficiently interesting. They have an aversion to work if it is at all routine, but they can apply themselves to tasks which are outside the run of the mill demands. In other words, the mind has lost its vitality, but it can be STIMULATED into activity when the person is properly motivated.

Generally, though, every day demands for mental exertion are too much for Calc. phos. patients. Unlike Calc. carb. patients, who will continue uncomplaining to do the mental tasks place infront of them, Calc. phos. will want to avoid them. Mental exertion may bring on a headache. It is a prime remedy to think of in school children who get headaches from mental exertion; by contrast, Calc. carb. is more indicated in school children who get headaches after PHYSICAL exertion.

Calc. phos. patients have ailments from grief or from bad news. Suppose a person receives a phone call saying that his son has been killed in a car accident. Most people would experience an acute spasm of grief, with shouting and weeping etc. and gradually the system would recover. The Calc. phos. patients, however, will be completely overwhelmed, he will collapse altogether, unable to cope with the situation in any way. It is not so much the grief *PER SE* that affects him; it is the sheer stress of the event

On the emotional level, there is a sluggishness which manifests as indifference or apathy. All motivation seems lost. This is not as severe as we see in Phosphoric acid, however. In Calc. phos.

the stillness is not so absolute; the person is still animated by a tremendous discontent.

Finally, on the physical level, the Calc. phos. patient experiences a loss of stamina. After a shock or some other stressful event, he notices that he connot play his customary game of tennis without getting out of breath or exhausted. Just as the mind has become flabby, so have the muscles.

The fundamental thing to remember about Calc. phos. is that this lack of vitality on mental, emotional, and physical levels produces a profound discontent in the person. He realises that something has gone wrong, but he doesn't know what he wants. He connot be stisfied by anything. This state can appear similar to Tuberculinum, but it has a completely different origin and does not have the maliciousness of Tuberculinum. It is closer to Chamomilla, but without the agressiveness and violence of Chamomilla.

The Calc. phos. image in children is helpful in understanding the situation in adults. I remember a doctor's child who had had a head injury. He became very peevish and irritable. We would ask, "What is wrong? Are you in pain? What do you want?" With each question, he only cried louder and louder. He used to wake up in the night screaming, but he could give no reason. The parents even took him outside for a walk at 3 a.m. but soon he was wailing again. Naturally, I tried Chamomilla in this case, but it did not work. Finally Calc. phos. cleared up the problem.

It is this discontent which characterises the adult state as well. They moan and groan and complain, but there is no way to satisfy them. They sense that something is deeply wrong in their organism, but they can find no way of correcting it. The discontent even penetrates their sleep; they moan in their sleep.

As with many remedies prepared from salts, Calc. phos. combines symptomatology from its components. It has the Calc. carb. aggravation from exertion (although not its endurance for mental exertion), but it has the Phosphorus ability to be stimulated into functioning. It has slowness in learning to talk or walk, like Calc. carb. Unique to Calc. phos., however, is slow closing of the fontanelles, and the "growing pains" of children due to slow closure of epiphyses.

Calcarea Phosphorica

The Phosphorus influence is strongly mainfest in a symptom I have observed to be cured in Calc. phos. patients; fear of thunderstorms. This symptom is not listed in Kent's Repertory, but it is so prominent in my experience that I have added it in the second degree. From experience, I would also add Calc. phos. to the rubrics, Sympathetic, and Anxiety about Others, Calc. phos. patients suffer with others, but with the difference that they are somewhat more detached than Phosphorus. In Calc. phos. it is more of an inward affair, less overtly giving then Phosphorus. Basically, Calc. phos. patients do not have the energy or motivation to give as much as Phosphorus patients.

Now, let me mention some of the key physical symptoms which distinguish Calc. phos. The primary target, of course, is the cervical region and the upper thoracic area, including the scapulae. There may be electric-like shocks which seem to explode in all directions. These pains are especially aggravated by drafts and cold wet weather—like Rhus tox and Cimicifuga.

The cervical region, in general, is an interesting region for studying remedies and various causations. On the mental/emotional level, specifically, pains in this area symbolise conflicts between perceived demands and doubt about the ability to meet those demands. Modern urban society particularly influences this conflict. Many stresses are applied with which our organisms are unaccustomed; if the vitality of an individual patient is unable to cope with these stresses, the defence mechanism creates a blockage in the cervical region, the conduit connecting the mental and emotional "organs" of the body. This process can occur with other remedies as well, but it is particularly prominent in the pathology of Calc. phos. It feels as if a hand is clutching the blood vessels of the neck and cutting off the circulation.

In general, of course, Calc. phos. is known to be intolerant to cold wet weather. This is especially so when the snow melts. The suffering may not be particularly severe while the snow is actually falling, but when it melts and the humidity rises, they become stiff all over.

It is true that Calc. phos. patients are generally intolerant to cold, but the Phosphorus element shows its influence again in an exceptional patient which can be warm blooded. Even in these exceptional patients, however, the LOCAL pains are still aggravated by cold wet weather. Also, even these patients have the cold feet which are typical in Calc. phos.

The stiffness in Calc. phos. can resemble Rhus tox in that it is aggravated in the morning and ameliorated by motion during the day. Ligaments and tendons in Calc. phos. seem to lose their vitality and elasticity. In particular, this allows the spine to lose its normal alignment. For this reason, Calc. phos. is one of the main remedies for scoliosis.

Sometimes Calc. phos. patients develop sighing which is similar to Ignatia. This might not necessarily occur after a grief. It is as if there is not enough oxygen, and the patient is compelled to take deep breaths which are not satisfying. Sometimes there is a cramping feeling in the solar plexus which is indistinguishable from Ignatia. In addition, there can be perspiration in the face, which is a keynote of Ignatia.

Calc. phos. has a desire for sweets, even though it is not listed in the Repertory. It also has a desire for smoked meats. such as salami.

An interesting observation I have made is that Calc. phos. is one remedy that tends to produce prolonged aggravations—even 10—20 days. It seems that it goes very deeply into the whole organism and stirs up many deep problems on the way toward cure. Calc. phos. is a very useful remedy—one that is irreplaceable when indicated.

CANNABIS INDICA (*cann-i.*)

Cannabis indica is a remedy which is certain to come into increasing use in our modern societies with their increasing use of psychoactive drugs. Naturally Cannabis is indicated in cases whose symptomatology is focussed in large part on the mental and emotional planes. It is interesting that there seems to be two basic types of people requiring Cannabis indica, each quite distinct from the other. One type is by nature a primarily emotional, ethereal person—someone who relates to things generally through the emotional realm rather than the mental. The other is primarily a mental type over stimulated in the mind, and governed by the fear of loss of control. I will discuss the symptomatologies of these two types separately.

The first, emotional type of person prefers not to use the mind. These people do not do mathematical or analytical tasks very well. As the Cannabis indica pathology overtakes them, they begin to feel light, ethereal and ecstatic. They seem to enjoy a blissful, floating state much of the time. They feel very light, not at all grounded—"spaced out".

These people seem to have a very tenuous connection between the vital body and the physical body. They seem to leave their body very easily. They easily experience *samadhi*–like states and trances, whether or not they are familiar with spiritual methods seeking such experiences. In these states they may readily experience psychic phenomena as well. On falling asleep, especially, they have the sensation of leaving the body and travelling in other dimensions. Sometimes they wake during the night and feel they are not in their body. During this state, they may try to make their legs move, and they find they cannot; they will them to move, but nothing happens. This is a cataleptic-like state, and it can be very frightening.

Most of the time these patients are in an ecstatic, exalted state, but when they feel the most separated from the body they become deeply terrified. They feel convinced that they can die in such a state—despite all reassurance to the contrary. Thus, they have a fear of death or a fear of insanity—but in these people the fearful states pass away in a short time.

These ethereal people also experience distortions of sensory perception. Cannabis indica speeds up all the senses. All impressions are received much more rapidly and vividly. Because of this increased intensity, time itself seems distorted. Internally, they feel very stimulated, so external events seem to happen more slowly than usual. This is the reason for the symptom "Time passes too slowly." Spatial distortions also occur. They feel that they are far removed from objects, that they are travelling or flowing away from things. Their limbs may seem to shrink in size. Again these feelings are manifestations of the easy etheric disconnection these people experience.

Despite their ecstasy, these people, in their conscious mind realise that this is a pathological state. The mind becomes hazy, vague, scattered. They become inefficient in their tasks, and they cannot focus on reality for any length of time. Typically these people drift from one job to another because of the dissatisfaction. They leave a job simply because they have lost interest; they prefer to do something else. They do not feel any bitterness about this. Indeed, they are mild, sweet people in general; they are very easy going.

It is this first type of Cannabis patients who laugh easily and immoderately at anything. Their emotional reactions are easily stimulated by external impressions.

Now, the second type—the mentalised Cannabis patients—are almost the complete opposite. These people are not at all happy or easy to get along with. They also have felt a sense of leaving the body—but only in certain parts. Certain parts seem to become light, as if they are floating away. This is especially felt in the extremities. The arm feels as if the bones are no longer there, and it becomes so light that it could float away.

To these mentalised Cannabis patients such sensations are terrifying. They are losing control of the arm; it is going its own way. Any loss of control creates tremendous anxiety and fear in them. These people feel a constant fear of insanity, which is another way of expressing a fear of losing control. Similarly, they may describe it as a fear of death. This anxiety state is continuous and motivates their behaviour to such a degree that you may consider remedies such as Phosphorus, Arsenicum, or Nitric

Cannabis Indica

acid. Also, this anxiety is generally felt in the stomach or in the chest.

Cannabis indica, especially in these mind-oriented patients seems to directly stimulate the brain. These people are constantly theorising about everything. They can be very interesting to talk to. They have their own ideas about what is happening in the world, about their own health, about various projects they are involved in, etc. Especially in our age of experimentation with various religions or spiritual approaches, these Cannabis patients are full of ideas about each practice. They are very quick and intelligent, and they can see anything from different angles at once.

Such patients may seem very educated and well-read, and in fact they often are, but they are not efficient in mental activities. Their minds are very scattered. Their theories have no beginning and no end; they are not verifiable because they are not grounded in reality. They jump from one idea to another, very much like Lachesis. At first, such patients may make you think of Lachesis, but as you listen further you realise how ungrounded their ideas are. Lachesis patients jump from one subject to another, but their ideas are more concrete and factual.

During a consultation, such a patient can pose great difficulty. They are very difficult to pin down. You may tell the patient, "Since you seem to have such a great thirst I can base my prescription on that symptom." Immediately, she will say, "Oh, wait a moment. I didn't mean THIRST exactly. I am sure that my thirst is really a desire for salt, because it must be caused by the sardines I ate a while ago. They must have thrown my system off." This kind of process occurs with every symptom until you feel you have nothing to go on. They see everything from so many angles and in such relative terms that they cannot be pinned down to anything definite.

Also, you might not realise the extent of their theorising during the course of the interview. They do not see it as a problem; indeed they may not even be aware of it. During the interview such a person talks only about heartburn or constipation, etc. Perhaps he did admit to some fear of death and excessive thirst, and you decide upon Arsenicum or Phosphorus. Then, during casual conversation after the interview, you bring up a few general subjects of conversation, and you suddenly discover that he is full of theories, mostly far-out in nature. Then Cannabis indica comes to mind.

In addition, these mentalised Cannabis patients are very critical. With each prescription or suggestion you make, they want to know exactly why you came to that particular decision. They must feel in complete control at all times; they are driven by their underlying fear of insanity. For this reason they are always challenging and questioning. They are difficult people—quite opposite from the easy going and happy first type of Cannabis patient.

Characteristically, Cannabis indica is extremely thirsty, expecially in acute situations. This, coupled with the fear of death, can lead to confusion with Arsenicum. There is one important differential point, however; Cannabis patients always want to rest and they feel better from lying down. Actually, from what I have observed, this is actually a mentalised symptom. They mentally arrive at the conclusion that they are better from lying down, and so that is what they do. If you force them to take a walk, especially in fresh air, they feel better. You must be careful not to over exert them, however; over exertion makes all Cannabis symptoms worse.

The mentalised type of Cannabis patients have very strong desires for sex. In maintaining control it seems that their energy becomes concentrated in the sexual sphere. The desire is so strong that if they do not have a partner available in the moment they will resort to masturbation. They are not particularly choosey about their partners; they just want quick satisfaction. Consequently they are quite susceptible to gonorrhoea. Cannabis is one of the remedies that could be indicated in acute gonorrhoea, although its yellow, thick discharge is of no value in the prescription because it is common in gonorrhoea; the characteristic mental picture would have to be present.

Cannabis indica has a variety of urinary symptom—it is often indicated in infections of the bladder, urethra, and kidneys. It is also indicated in certain early neurological cases characterised by weakness and numbness of the extremities—prior to the stage of true paralysis or actual clinical diagnosis.

Cannabis indica probably has a usefulness in patients who have had a so-called "Bad trip" which has left a lasting effect on the mental sphere. This would be true whether the bad experience occurred on hashish itself, or LSD, mescaline, heroin, or others. It may also be needed in people whose constitutions have broken down into a dull, hazy, scattered mental state after using many such drugs over a period of years. If the mental state has become severely dulled, Phosphoric acid would be the first remedy to consider, but Cannabis indica and Agnus castus would be others to remember.

NOSTALGIA OF THE PAST

CAPSICUM ANNUUM (*caps.*)

- More often men than women.
- 2 STAGES—which have common and opposing characteristics.
- Type is obese, flabby, redness in face and especially nose. Drunkards nose and face (similar Aeculus). The flabbiness is unique—very thick, feels stomach is a sac without any fibre, least food blows it up, can put on 10 kg. in 1 week—may confuse with Kali bich.
- Low vitality, easily tired, feel cold, get obese (Calc. carb.—which will make more obese and increase appetite, easily confused; Ferrum met; white with pale cheeks.)
- Very sensitive, feel easily insulted, insecure without social relationship, not withdrawn like Nat. mur., tries to be more sociable to hide insecurity.
- NOSTALGIA—** emotions go back to past events with such force that it overtakes the whole person and he thinks he will die—can't stand it. Lives totally in the past.
- If away from home, has to go back home.
- Guilt, fear of police though they have done nothing (Nat. carb., Merc.)
- When reaches point where can't tolerate past emotions, he switches off completely, and "Can't" or won't remember, no feelings left. This is not the indifference of Phos. ac. or the dead feeling of Carbo veg.
- Tremendous feeling of anxiety always there (hidden). Has to accomplish something, but the mind is dull, and anxious because cannot accomplish what he has to do.
- Feels exposed to the insults of others.

SLEEP: Tired, falls asleep immediately. Wakes after 3 hours and overtaken by anxiety and insecurity. Stays awake 2 hours, then falls asleep again until late morning.

IN SECOND STAGE

- Desire for stimulation which < –coffee, beer, whisky, pepper salt, but does not crave.

Capsicum Annuum

- May be irritable and awkward but desire security.
- Lazy, try to do best with least effort.
- Lies in unusual position on back with right knee raised to get to sleep.
- Ulcers, haemorrhoids, palpitations, anxiety, depression.
- No fear of death.
- Remedy usually given after failure of others (e.g. Calc, Nux).
- The organism is lazy, difficult to arouse.
- Awkward (not as much as Apis, Bovista).
- Fear of censure.
- Homesick with red cheeks.
- In children, great obstinacy and capriciousness (Cham, Cina).
- Sensitive to noise during chill.
- Enlarged sensation in head.
- Pain in head during coughing.
- *Severe mastoiditis with burning pain.
- Lack of reflection.
- *Anxiety is not easily seen (Opposite of Helleborus).
- Add to Repertory for desires pepper.

EAR : Mastoiditis severe and burning. Hearing becomes acute during a chill.
MOUTH : Ulcers, burning, gums inflamed.
COUGH : ** Offensive odour from coughing, even to patient himself.
THROAT : Red. Hoarse from over-use of voice.
- Coffee causes nausea (but desires it).
- Thirst before chill. *Thirst after stool.
* BLADDER : Pain during coughing. Used in gonorrhoea with creamy discharge.
- Sensation of cold air in rectum.
GENITALIA : Cold in morning on waking.
- Sleeplessness from homesickness.
GENERAL : > emotion, warmth.
            < cold, stimulants.
N.B. Capsicum wakes 3 hours after going to sleep whatever time this may be, i.e. not a specific time like Kali bich.

[Handwritten notes: HYPERACTIVITY / IDEALISTIC ANARCHISTS / SLOWLY LOSING MENTAL POWER]

CAUSTICUM HAHNEMANNI (caust.)

[Handwritten note: AGGRAVATED BY COLD WEATHER]

The main idea permeating Causticum is GRADUAL PARALYSIS following an initial phase of excessive hypersensitivity and over-reactivity. This concept runs through all levels of Cuasticum's existence—mental, emotional and physical. In general, the primary target of Causticum pathology is the central and peripheral nervous system.

From this essence, it is easy to imagine the type of people who tend to eventually acquire Causticum symptomatology; sensitive people, who are easily excitable, quick to react; they absorb all impressions from the environment, responding with hyperactivity and over-reaction, particularly in those functions governed by the nervous system.

Causticum people possess a strong sense of social justice, which manifests in particular as intolerance to any kind of authority. It is interesting in this regard to contrast Causticum with Staphysagria, which are complementary to one another. Staph. accepts authority to an extreme degree; he will not be able to confront anybody, even to stand up for his own rights. Causticum is exactly the opposite. He will not tolerate anything that oppresses either himself or others. Even in the early stages prior to development of florid pathology, one can detect the Causticum tendency in a person by this excessive sensitivity to oppressive influences, combined with excessive excitability of the central nervous system. Once the person's health has declined to a more pathological degree, this tendency becomes exaggerated to the point where the patient would perhaps best be described as anarchistic. Such people are easily and deeply hurt, because injustice and oppressions can be found in almost every circumstance of life. They are anarchists of the idealistic kind; very sincere and earnest, and therefore vulnerable.

When such people have been through many disappointments, griefs and vexations, the initial state of over-reactivity becomes turned inward. Whereas the patient was extroverted, revolutionary activist, these energies become focused inward.

Causticum Hahnemanni

It is as if they are cramping him inside. They cause him to withdraw, and the resulting pathology gradually weakens the mental, emotional, and physical levels. At first, he wants to destroy the outside world because it is not what it should be. With time, however, he finds himself bound up by diminished nervous system reflexes, hardened and shortened tendons, and a general state of inflexibility.

The main characteristic of Caustiucum throughout this process is that of GRADUALITY. It is not a state which comes on suddenly. It takes a long time for the initial over-reactivity to invert itself into the state of cramped paralysis of function.

As a general rule, the nervous system, muscles, and connective tissue manifest symptoms first. Causticum is a prominent remedy to consider in patients suffering from locomotor ataxia, myopathy, multiple sclerosis, or myasthenia of gradual onset, a very characteristic feature of Causticum is paralysis of LOCAL organs. There may be facial paralysis, paralysis or dysfunction of the oesophagus, uncontrolled drooping of the upper eyelids, stammering from dysfunction of the tongue, biting of the cheeks while talking or chewing, dysfunction of bladder sphincter mucles, and paralysis of the extremities.

The nervous system vulnerability also manifests in another way. If a Causticum patient suppresses a skin eruption with a strong ointment such as zinc or cortisone, the suppression progresses directly into the nervous system, and often into deeper mental or emotional states.

Gradually, the inversion of hyper-activity into hypo-active states reaches into the mental/emotional planes. More and more he has forebodings that something terrible is going to happen to him or to his relatives. Slowly, he develops other fears as well; fear of the dark, fear of being alone especially at night, and a fear of dogs.

While he was healthy, the Causticum patient's mental faculties were very acute. Whereas he once was very intellectual person; philosophising, analysing things deeply and with great capacity—he starts feeling that he is losing his mental power and slowly sliding into a state of imbecility. This is not an animated kind of insanity, of course; it is a passive state. His mental faculties become completely paralysed in the final stage.

Again it needs to be emphasised that this is a gradual decline. At first, the patient begins to notice a lessening of mental powers, then comes the foreboding that something bad is going to happen to him or others, next other fears begin to manifest, and finally the degeneration into passive imbecility.

It is well known that Causticum is a highly sympathetic remedy. This sympathy may not be prominent in the early stages of stimulation but the prescriber can detect the tendency underneath. The excessive concern for injustices in the world, and intolerance to authority, are the early signs which MANIFEST LATER as extreme sympathy for the pain of others. For example, I recall a woman in labour who could not tolerate the cries and screams of other women in labour. Despite the fact that the ward was very hot, she had to close the doors and windows tight in order to avoid hearing the sufferings of the other women.

On the physical level, Causticum has a variety of quite characteristic symptoms to guide or confirm a prescription. The most characteristic modality is AGGRAVATION BY DRY COLD WEATHER. Exposure to dry cold air can immediately affect the nervous system, especially peripherally. Paralysis may date from exposure to cold, affecting facial muscles, vocal cords (complete aphonia, especially in the morning). Peculiarly enough, there is an amelioration of rheumatic pains in wet weather—even in cold wet. On the other hand, the rheumatic pains are strikingly aggravated by BATHING in cold water, while DRINKING cold water ameliorates gastritis pains and especially the cough (ALTHOUGH NOT AS DRAMATICALLY AS THE AMELIORATION FROM COLD DRINKS IN THE Spongia cough).

The pains of Causticum are quite characteristic. In the paralytic state, there are characteristic electric-like shooting pains in the affected area. Alumina and Arg. nit. are more commonly indicated for these kinds of pains, but Causticum should not be forgotten. Of course, there are all kinds of cramping pains and muscle twitching in Causticum. There are convulsions, chorea, torticollis, and a peculiar kind of nervous restlessness of the legs especially while lying in bed.

Another type of Causticum pain is a feeling of RAWNESS, "like an open wound." This is most characteristic during bronchitis. The patient suffers from a powerful cough accompanied by a raw pain in the chest, causing him to hold his chest while coughing. Causticum has a desire for salt and an aversion to sweets. This is one of the very few remedies that displays this combination. It also has a peculiar desire for smoked meat (along with Tuberculinum, Kreosotum, and Calc. phos.).

The most characteristic skin symptoms, found in Causticum are warts, particularly warts on the face and on the fingers near the nails. Causticum should always be considered for such warts, along with Thuja and Lac caninum. Fissures of the intertriginous areas and anus are also well known in Causticum. Typical Causticum eruptions are found around the nose, inside and outside the wings of the nose, and on the tip of the nose, (if there is an eruption on the tip of the nose, Aethusa should also be remembered).

Causticum is one remedy not to forget in hay fever when there is itching inside or outside the wings of the nose, there is sneezing upon waking in the morning, a viscid catarrh drips from the postnasal membranes. In hay fever, one of the most characteristic symptoms of Causticum is obstruction of the nose while lying down, especially at night.

Because the mucous is very viscid, the patient gets the feeling that it has stuck low in the trachea and cannot be brought up even by continuous coughing. This is similar to Medorrhinum, which, however, has the sensation of the mucous being stuck higher up in the trachea.

The Causticum cough is typically a hollow, deep cough of great force. It is, therefore, not surprising that it is usually accompanied by loss of urine. In CAUSTICUM, LOSS OF URINE WILL BE FOUND WITH ANY pressure on the urinary bladder, whether from sneezing, laughing or coughing.

When the nerve supply to the bladder is paralysed, there may be either retention of urine or involuntary loss of urine. If the muscles of expulsion are affected, urine is retained sometimes resulting in extensive stretching of the bladder wall. Kent provides a memorable description of this circumstance; "A woman who is too greatly embarrassed to pass through a crowd of observing men to the closet at the end of a railroad car, at the end of the journey finds that she is unable to pass the urine. Retention of urine from straining the muscles of the bladder. If the patient

MUSCLE PARALYSIS REMEDIES

is chilled at the time, the remedy may be Rhus. Rhus and Causticum are the two great remedies for paralytic weakness of muscles from being overstrained, or from being overstrained and chilled.

On the other hand, there may be a loss of sensation in the urethra, causing the patient to lose urine invloluntarily without being aware of it. This is why Causticum is one of the leading remedies in childhood enuresis.

As the whole organism gradually declines into a paralytic state, there may be a decrease of sexual urge and pleasure. Causticum is one of the main remedies for frigidity in women—along with others, of course, like Sepia, Graphites, Natrum mur. etc.

In summary, Causticum is characterised by gradual changes, beginning with an initial hyper-reactivity, sensitivity to injustice and authority, and anarchism; this progresses to paralysis of the neuromuscular system, fears and forebodings and finally decline into passive imbecility. The primary traget of pathology is the nervous system, which shows paralysis accompanied by initial phases of cramping and twitching, and electric shock-like pains in the affected part. Characteristic confirmatory symptoms include aggravation from dry cold, desire for salt and smoked meat, aversion to sweets, warts on the face and fingers, retention or loss of urine, and a deep hollow cough with viscid mucous low in the trachea.

CARBO VEGETABILIS (carb-v.)

Carbo veg. is a remedy which has been well described in our books. Especially in its acute aspect, one is unlikely to miss it. There are three primary characteristics which constitute the essence of Carbo veg. First, there is a general SLUGGISHNESS of the organism, especially in the circulation but also of the emotions and mind. This then is coupled with COLDNESS which runs throughout the body—coldness of the breath, of the nose, of the face, of the extremities. This coldness, however, is accompanied by a strong DESIRE TO BE FANNED.

In Carbo veg. it is frequently the case that the health is affected by the shock of an acute illness (usually pneumonia) or an accident. The overall vitality is lowered by a notch ever since an accident; thus, Arnica is not always the appropriate remedy for this situation. You may study such a case and discover that there are too few symptoms to prescribe any other remedy but you see coldness, weakness and emotional indifference. This is enough to prescribe Carbo veg. In many of the books, it is said that Carbo veg. is prescribed after an illness or accident, but one should not develop a routine of this. If the patient is warmblooded and vital but suffers some problem since experiencing a shock, do not give Carbo veg. The sluggishness which affects the physical level also characterises the emotional plane. There is indifference; the patient does not care whether he lives or dies. This apathy is somewhat like that of Phosphoric acid. The patient may be given good news but is incapable of feeling cheerful about it. Even after bad news, he or she says, "It doesn't matter".

Sluggishness on the mental level manifests as DULLNESS of the mind. The mind is slow to comprehend. The patient cannot concentrate, cannot do the usual work. Because the mind is not functioning properly, there is indecision or irresolution. This mental condition seems to result from inadequate oxygenation of the brain. The circulation is sluggish, so not enough oxygen reaches the brain.

It is interesting that there are SPELLS of loss of memory in Carbo veg. The patient SUDDENLY loses his memory for a time, but it later returns just as suddenly. Again, it is as if the circulation were temporarily compromised.

Carbo veg. may get fixed ideas—"arterio-sclerotic" ideas. A woman may read in a magazine that butter is bad for health and she insists on this idea in an inflexible manner. There can be no exceptions to the rule. She wil not change her opinion. It is as if there is not enough vitality in the brain to understand any other point of view.

Carbo veg. may not affect all three levels in any given individual. It is primarily a physical remedy, with relatively minor manifestations on deeper levels. In my experience, it is rare to encounter a Carbo veg. patient who is mentally ill.

On the physical level, Carbo veg. can affect any system, but its primary actions are on the venous circulation, the digestive tract, and the respiratory system. When the symptoms occur in the respiratory tract, it primarily affects the LOWER tract. It becomes indicated when lung conditions have progressed to a fairly advanced state. There may be a sudden decline from pneumonia. Or a particular type of asthma develops—aggravated by lying down and relieved by vigorous fanning.

The modality, aggravation from lying down is easy to understand in Carbo veg. in light of the sluggishness. The blood seems to stagnate when the patient lies down. The headache becomes intolerable. The respiration feels as if it has been arrested, especially when falling asleep or during sleep. The patient jumps up from bed suddenly, like Lachesis. It is as if there is inadequate tonus in the veins to equilibrate the circulation. The usual automatic mechanisms whereby the circulation adjusts to changes of position are sluggish.

The acute condition of Carbo veg. is unmistakeable. You may have been treating a pneumonia case, but progress has been slow. Suddenly the patient goes into a state of collapse, with laboured breathing, coldness of extremities, coldness of the breath, coldness of the tongue, and coldness of the nose. The body temperature drops. The colour becomes a deathly white, with blueness around the lips and on the tips of the fingers. The patient appears like a corpse, and she feels like life is leaving her! She does not

Carbo Vegetabilis

fear death; indeed, she may even desire it. She feels so indifferent that it doesn't seem worth while to continue. Once you see this death-like state coming on suddenly, you cannot miss Carbo veg.

You may have another patient suffering from severe forcible vomiting. You give Chelidonium, Veratrum album or Arsenicum, but the patient suddenly becomes white with blueness in areas of least circulation, becomes covered with cold perspiration, the body temperature drops, and the breath becomes cold. The patient goes into a faint. This is a picture of Carbo veg. and you may observe a dramatic amelioration from its administration.

Carbo veg. is used more often as an acute remedy than as a deep constitutional, but there are nevertheless some constitutional indications. It is often indicated in digestive disorders—extreme bloatendness, peptic ulcer, gastritis, colitis. The bloatedness can be very extreme and continuous, with frequent eructations which relieve. This condition is aggravated by overeating in general, and specifically by fat or butter. The bloatedness causes the diaphragm to press on the heart and thus causes periodic collapses. Such a patient may eat a large meal and drink a little wine, and then the pressure of the diaphragm causes the patient to faint even at the table.

Even though the bloatedness is often caused by overeating, do not get the impression that the Carbo veg. patient is obese. This may be so, but the more usual appearance is of a thin patient.

Carbo veg. may be indicated in very old people with indolent ulcers. They have ulcers that do not heal and degenerate into a gangrenous condition. Other remedies that may have this condition are Lachesis, Hepar sulphur, Calcarea carbonica and Carbo animalis, but Carbo veg. particularly fits the very elderly—those over, say, 80 years of age—who are cold, bloated and intolerant to fat.

In addition to intolerance to fat, Carbo veg. is intolerant to alcohol. There may not necessarily be a strong reaction, but enough that the patient notices it. Even after just a sip of alcohol, there may be flushing of the face, or the face may be pale but the patient feels weak inside.

The desire to be fanned is a striking keynote characteristic for Carbo veg. This manifests particularly during the acute state—in collapse or during dyspnoea. Carbo veg. does not merely desire fresh air alone but wants a forceful wind blowing on the face. He may even tell you that if he becomes short of breath while in a moving car, he will stick his head out of the window. If someone is fanning a Carbo veg. patient, the fanning must be very fast and forceful. It is as if the patient is trying to inject oxygen into the system.

Comparison of remedies that desire fresh air or fanning provides an excellent study in the high degree of individualisation needed in homoeopathy. As we take cases and repertorise the totality of symptoms, it is easy to fall into the trap of merely matching data. However, even within each particular rubric, one needs to know precisely which states individualise one remedy (patient) from another. Arsenicum, for example, is a cold remedy that desires fresh air; Arsenicum does not want the body exposed at all, but the head is relieved by cool air. Even so, Arsenicum never want a strong wind blowing on the face as does Carbo veg. Of course, warmblooded remedies like Pulsatilla are often aggravated in a warm stuffy room and want fresh air but in Pulsatilla it is merely a need to be cooled. Apis is a warmblooded remedy that wants to be fanned, but Apis is content with gentle fanning. The most warmblooded remedy of all, Secale, needs to be fanned very aggressively, not so much because of the need for oxygen, but because of the need for relief from the internal heat.

The opposite situation, aggravation from wind, is also instructive of the need for individualisation. Many remedies have an aversion to wind, but specifically for what reason? Lycopodium, of course, enjoys being outdoors in the fresh air, but feels bad whenever directly exposed to wind. Nux vomica can be aggravated even by being indoors while wind is blowing outside, in Nux vomica this is an aggravation of the mental state specifically. Rhododendron also has an aggravation from wind blowing outdoors, but this is caused by the corresponding electormagnetic changes in the atmosphere. All of Rhododendron's physical complaints are stirred up—he feels on edge, his muscles become stiff, he may become irritable, like Nux, but because of the pains.

As mentioned earlier Carbo veg. is intolerant to fat and butter. There is a characteristically strong desire for salt and a lesser desire for sweets and coffee.

Carbo Vegetabilis

Carbo veg. affects the physical level most strongly, but it may affect the emotional level to some degree. There are few anxieties of fears of any strength. There is no fear of death, which helps to differentiate Carbo veg. from Arsenicum or Phosphorus. It may have some anxiety about health, especially when closing the eyes on bed at night, but not nearly so prominently as in other remedies. Interestingly, Carbo veg. does not have a fear of the dark, but it is AGGRAVATED by darkness. Carbo veg. may have a fear of ghost, like Lycopodium. Also, just as Carbo veg. can be ill since the shock of an accident, it also has a characteristic fear of accidents.

Carbo veg. is complementary to Arsenicum and Phosphorus. Patients who have responded well to these remedies sometimes experience great relief from their anxieties, but then the disease focusses on the digestive tract and causes severe bloatedness. They forget about their old fears and anxieties althogether and focus their attention solely on the bloatedness. This is a situation in which Carbo veg. is likely to follow well.

Lycopodium can be easily confused with Carbo veg. Both have tremendous bloatedness and eructations, but Carbo veg. is more readily relieved by the eructations than Lycopodium. Lycopodium is not as severely cold as Carbo veg. Carbo veg. has a strong desire for salt and less desire for sweets; Lycopodium has the opposite. The position of sleep can be helpful; Carbo veg. needs to sleep propped up, whereas Lycopodium prefers to sleep on the right side. As mentioned, Lycopodium benefits by being in fresh air, but is actually aggravated by direct wind. Finally, Carbo veg. does not have the strong morning aggravation that is seen in Lycopodium.

NEED TO DOMINATE
REALISTIC ANXIETY (ABOUT HEALTH)

CHELIDONIUM MAJUS (chel.)

In my experience Chelidonium is quite similar in its constitutional picture to Lycopodium. The two can be quite dificult to differentiate, especially when you consider the whole person.

In my observation Chelidonium patients are quite FORCEFUL individuals. They seem to have a need to dominate others. They are very opinionated, and they want to force their opinions onto others, even with all good intentions. They have a definite sense of what is right and wrong even in fields outside their own area of expertise. They are quick to give advice, and then feel insulted if their opinions are not followed. In this respect, Chelidonium is similar to Dulcamara.

This dictatorial aspect of Chelidonium is reminiscent of Lycopodium, of course, but there is a fundamental difference. Lycopodium is fundamentally a coward and therefore limits his domination to those whom he can control-subordinates childern, etc. Chelidonium is not a coward and does not change behaviour depending upon who he is speaking to. He will force his opinions on superiors just as readily as upon subordinates. Chelidonium does not have the pacifism seenin most other liver remedies. Such a patient will not hesitata to fight for his or her own rights or opinions. prod-

In a sense, Chelidonium patients are concerned about others, but this is not an anxiety about others which arises out of a human sensitivity. It is more of a guilty feeling. They will make great sacrifices for someone, but at the same time they will not hesitate to make critical remarks in the presence of the same person, and if the other person does not follow their advice, they will at first be insulted and then quickly lose interest in that person. Their orientation is more toward "getting the job done" than truly understanding and serving another's needs.

It seems that there is a kind of deep insecurity which leads Chelidonium patients to help and dominate others. They are strong willed people, and they seem to derive a sense of security and satisfaction out of getting other to do their bidding.

In particular, Chelidonium patients develop a strong attachment

Chelidonium Majus

to one specific person—a husband or a wife, for example. They have then considerable anxiety about the well-being of that particular person. It is in this respect that Chelidonium should be added to the rubric. Anxiety about others. Even so, a Chelidonium woman, for instance, who is greatly attached to her husband will not hesitate to dominate him. She may be so forceful in her personality that the husband simply shuts up and lets her do all the talking.

Chelidonium patients are realists. They are very matter of fact and hard headed. They are definitely not intellectuals; indeed they may be anti-intellectual. Whenever possible, they tend to shun intellectual work, mathematical problems, abstractions, etc. They would never "waste" time analysing their emotions, explaining situations, interpreting behaviour, etc. One could even describe Chelidonium patients as mentally indolent—apathetic and lazy.

Chelidonium patients are not easily overtaken by their emotions. They are not at all sentimental. They do not easily express affection. However, they do expect others to display tenderness and affection toward them.

On the emotional plane, Chelidonium patients can have anxieties—anxieties about someone to whom they are attached, and also anxiety about their own health. This anxiety about health may not be as strong as it is in other remedies, but it is definitely present. In Chelidonium this is a realistic anxiety. These patients will have check-up by the most qualified doctors, then, if there is even some slight problem they become anxious and want something practical and tangible to be done right away. In addition, they tend to be suspicious about what is being done. If the doctor diagnoses colitis the Chelidonium patient will not be satisfied. He asks, "Are you sure? Could it not be the liver, or the spleen? Have you considered all the possibilities?" His anxiety drives him to cover all bases.

Chelidonium patients also can experience deep depressions, but usually only briefly and over relatively minor matters. A Chelidonium woman may be very demanding of her husband, and then when he does not respond exactly the way she wishes, she broods and falls into a deep depression. But the next day she is over it and remains cheerful until the next minor disappointment occurs.

Chelidonium of course, is predominantly a liver remedy. A patient who has been suffering from Chelidonium symptomatology for some time will have a dirty yellowish hue to the skin, or even a copperish colour.

Like other liver remedies, Chelidonium's symptoms are characteristically worse in the morning. There is unrefreshed sleep. Also, Chelidonium has a specific time aggravation at 4 a.m., particularly regarding neuralgias and headaches. This is an interesting peculiarity considering the Lycopodium has a 4 p.m. aggravation. Chelidonium is not worse specifically in the afternoon, but both Chelidonium and Lycopodium feel better in the evening—after 8 p.m. or so.

Generally, Chelidonium patients are aggravated by cold, except the headaches, sinusitis, and neuralgias, which are ameliorated by cold. Chelidonium is characteristically worse from changes of weather even from cold to warm. It is known to be aggravated in general by wet weather, but I do not believe this is a strong symptom; I have seen several Chelidonium patients who are able to live near the sea with little difficulty.

Chelidonium is a markedly right-sided remedy. Especially during hepatitis pains, it has characteristic pain in the right hypochondrium which extends to the inferior angle of the scapula. In acute cases, this symptom is practically a necessity for prescribing Chelidonium. Chelidonium is not ameliorated by lying on the painful side.

Chelidonium has arthritic pains which are secondary to liver disease. These typically affect the right shoulder and both knees (with some preference for the right knee). The knee pains are markedly aggravated by walking. Chelidonium is one of the primary remedies to consider in knee pains aggravated by walking.

Chelidonium has a strong characteristic which I have not seen emphasised in the books. It has a strong desire for milk and milk products, especially cheese. It can have either a desire for or an aversion to cheese, but it is seldom neutral. In addition, Chelidonium desires warm drinks and warm food—and is made better by them.

Chelidonium develops slowly in its pathology, and is slow to respond once the remedy has been given. Do not be in a hurry to change remedies if the response after a month is not impressive (in a chronic case). Aside from the slowness of response, Chelidonium patients are unlikely to report improvement anyway. They are never satisfied until they see tangible, objective, incontrovertible results. Even if the remedy were to produce a miraculous change, such a patient will not admit it until a year or so of relief has passed. Even then he may be suspicious. He will say, "You say I am better, but the other doctors all said my liver will never be normal again. How can what you say be possible?" He may even insist on getting liver function tests in the hope that one of them will prove to you that the liver is still affected —all this in spite of relief.

Of course, differentiation between Lycopodium and Chelidonium can be quite a problem in a particular case. Generally, Chelidonium is much more forceful and heedless of risks in expressing his domineering opinions; Lycopodium is more timid and cowardly, limiting his domination to subordinates. Both have an anxiety about health, it is less intense and more realistic and matter of fact in Chelidonium. Both remedies are right-sided but Chelidonium's pain more characteristically radiates to the inferior angle of the scapula. Lycopodium tends to lie on its right side, whereas Chelidonium is not ameliorated in this position and will tend to lie on the left side. Both have bloatedness and distension but Chelidonium not nearly as intensely as Lycopodium. Lycopodium has much stronger desire for sweets than Chelidonium. Lycopodium usually is neutral about cheese, whereas Chelidonium either has a strong desire for or strong aversion to cheese. Both desire warm drinks and warm food and are ameliorated by them. Both do not feel well on waking, but Chelidonium has a specific aggravation at 4 a.m. Chelidonium does not share Lycopodium's specific 4 p.m. aggravation, but both remedies are ameliorated in the evening.

The differentiation between Chelidonium and Lycopodium is a perfect example of the necessity for underlining in recording cases. The differentiation is based mostly on shades of intensity, rather than black and white differences. It could be impossible to decide based upon a written case with no underlining to convey the intensity of the symptoms as described by the patient. Homoeopathy is a science based upon finely tuned shades of differences from one remedy another to. Perhaps nowhere else is this fact so evident as in comparing Chelidonium and Lycopodium.

Handwritten annotations at top:
- INSISTENT UPON OWN OPINIONS
- ANXIETY FOR OTHERS
- SCOPA NEL CULO
- EXAGGERATION

DULCAMARA (*dulc.*)

This chapter will focus mostly on the mental and emotional state of Dulcamara, since other Materia Medicas adequately describe the physical level. This material should be considered tentatively as it comes from my own observations and deductions based primarily on indepth experiences of two cases in particular which illustrate the essence of the remedy. Both patients happened to be women, but this should not imply that Dulcamara is a female remedy. It is interesting that, as one would expect from the provings, I had prescribed such remedies as Calc. carb., Rhus tox, and Kali carb. before settling on Dulcamara in these cases. It is only by careful examination of such illustrations in our practices that we can begin to paint the portrait of the true essence of a remedy.

Both of these women have very forceful, strong-willed personalities. They were DOMINEERING and POSSESSIVE in their relationship with other people, especially those closest to them. Dulcamara patients are very opinionated, insistent upon their own point of view, and then feel unappreciated when those around them do not show the gratitude they expect.

The typical Dulcamara patient carves out a territory, a sphere of influence—usually with her own family, but possibly including neighbours and friends as well. Within this sphere of influence she attempts to dominate others by her strong will and forceful opinions. She lives vicariously through others by trying to govern and control their lives.

Outside her own circle, however, she is suspicious of others. She is on guard. She becomes so wrapped up in her own state that she finds fault with other people. She expects that they will not understand her, that they will misunderstand and misinterpret her feelings and behaviour. During the initial interview she is very closed; she is willing to talk only about her concrete symptoms—her frequent colds, her hay fever, or her joint pains. She is unwilling to reveal more of herself until she is assured that the prescriber understands and appreciates her to her own satisfaction. One patient even changed doctors because she was convinced that he did not understand her. He did nothing specific to offend her, but she said she would never go back to him; she reported, "He is a nice person, but he does not understand me," merely because he was not forceful enough in backing up her own opinions.

This type of patient is very insistent upon her own point of view. She is always right, and she expects others to acknowledge that. During the interview in usual fashion, you listen quietly and sympathetically to what she has to say; you do not reply, but merely write down the symptoms in detail as she gives them to you. She wants you to believe her absolutely, however, so she feels unappreciated. When you begin to realise this, you reassure her that you do indeed believe what she is saying. She is very suspicious. It takes a lot of serious reassurance on your part to gain her confidence enough for her to open up and describe her true state.

Arising out of the Dulcamara patient's possessiveness is great anxiety about others. Her husband may be facing an important meeting at work, and she feels compelled to give him detailed instructions on how to behave, what to say, etc. This is not merely helpful advice, as Phosphorus might offer. Dulcamara insists that her opinions be followed, and she is disturbed if they are not. She insists that her son not marry, or if he does he must marry the woman of her choice. She is a busy body. She suffocates others in her domination and possessiveness.

The Dulcamara state, as you can see, is very self-centred. It almost never crosses her mind that others also have rights and freedom of choice. She is tremendously attached to those around her. She demands that they do exactly what SHE wants.

In Dulcamara, the anxiety for others is an anxiety for the health of her relatives in particular. This may be carried to such an extreme that she exaggerates trifles out of all proportion to reality. Little problems loom so large that they seem to create in her a kind of madness. This state is similar to Calc. carb., but if you inquire into the meaning of her exaggerations you discover that it arises fundamentally out of her possessiveness.

During her interview, to take a concrete example, the Dulcamara patient may report to you with great forcefulness and anxiety that her husband has a runny nose. She seems so obsessed by this that she seems to pass off her own problems. You cannot see why such a trivial problem means so much to her, but it does. Little things create an agony for her, a deep despair.

A Dulcamara patient's husband may have many things on his mind and leaves for work without saying goodbye. She then ruminates about this; "I have devoted my whole life to him, cooked for him, kept his clothes cleaned and pressed, and no he doesn't even take notice of me!" To take another example, after all her exhortations, her son leaves home and marries a woman not of her own choice. She feels unappreciated and falls into deep despair. Finally, she may even have suicidal thoughts. She says to herself, "I don't want to live any more."

Considering these complaints,. you have difficulty understanding her upset, so you inquire, "What is the problem? You have a nice family, your husband provides you with a nice home, your son is getting married to someone he loves. What is the trouble?" It is that she feels that they are all ungrateful. She tries to possess them, and they go their own way. This makes her feel—and appear—very "uptight". UPTIGHTNESS is very characteristic of Dulcamara, and you may even discover that this state has gone so far as to produce idiopathic hypertension. Dulcamara is an excellent remedy for high blood pressure in patients of this type.

Once someone leaves her circle of influence, the Dulcamara patient may continue to try to prove that her view was correct all along. Spitefully, she describes the terrible way her son is treated by his wife; "His wife doesn't cook for him, doesn't keep house properly. He is living in a terrible state!" Not knowing better, you may imagine that, he is living in a hovel. But if you happen to visit his home, you see immediately how much the patient has exaggerated the situation. You witness a well-kept, happy home, but the patient has picked up on minor faults and blown them out of proportion—merely in order to prove herself right.

The physical picture of Dulcamara, of course, is well described in all the books. Changes of weather from hot to cold brings on diarrhoea, joint pains, or coryza. It sometimes is a valuable remedy in hay fever. A prominent characteristic is the tremendous headache which comes on after a catarrh has been suppressed. It also has eruptions of the face, and if these are suppressed a painful facial neuralgia may occur.

When you first study a Dulcamara case, you may immediately think of Calc. carb., and indeed Dulcamara is quite similar in many respects. Dulcamra patients tend to be obese. They are chilly—particularly aggravated in changes from warm to cold. They may desire sweets. For years I puzzled over this dilemma, especially when Calcarea did not help much. I still cannot recall how Dulcamara came to mind, but it probably was triggered by some relatively minor physical symptoms. It is only after seeing Dulcamara dramatically transform a few cases like this that I could finally discern the beginning of its essence. After taking dulcamara these patients become much calmar, their blood pressure normalises, and they lose their extreme concern for their relatives.

Kali. carb. is another remedy that comes easily to mind in such cases. It is uptight, intolerant to cold and has a desire for sweets. Kali.carb. however, is much more independent than Dulcamara-not nearly so likely to be concerned about others.

Arsenicum, of course, is another remedy to compare. It has great anxiety about others and is chilly as well. Arsenicum, however, is anxious about losing his or her relatives because of dependency. He or she needs others to provide a feeling of security. Dulcamara's anxiety is just the opposite; it arises out of a sense of possessiveness, a need to dominate. In addition, Dulcamara is far more strong-willed and forceful than Arsenicum.

INSENSITIVE EXC. FOR OTHERS SUFFERENCE
ONLY UNDERSTANDS MATERIAL HELP
SLEEPING DISORDERS
MAINLY MALE CASES

FLUORICUM ACIDUM (fl-ac.)

THE CONSTITUTIONAL PICTURE

- Mainly a male remedy.
- A materialist—a man of the world.
- Enjoy life to its full extent—not bothered about spiritual development, awareness, discipline, etc.
- Crude energy—makes itself known early in life by a driving force for sexual intercourse. Often begins at age 13–14 and has to have sex every day.
- Not easy to discern. May come with falling of hair, or sleeplessness, or anxiety beyond their control. First few prescriptions do not do anything, then as you get to know them a better picture emerges.
- Early intercourse. Then early but short marriage. Then frequent change of relationship, but no satisfaction. Beautiful girl friends ; but superficial relationships. Do not care about inner relationship.
- Insensitive and aggressive. Not refined, do not understand sensitivity.
- Develop a feeling of superiority which is seen by actions to put down others e.g. will get all girl friends to wear blue shirts.
- Kind on another level. Like to help others materially—don't understand any other kind of help.
- Noon best time for sex 1-2 p.m.
- No real contact with others.
- Promote their own feeling of enjoyment.
- Cannot relate to wife and children if they don't please him.
- But very sensitive to suffering of others—will go to extremes to save the life of a child with cancer. This is because very deep down there is an anxiety about own health. Tremendous fear of cancer; as if exercise cancer by helping others.
- Tremendous fear of suffering—make friends with doctors. Want to enjoy life and die without suffering.

Fluoricum Acidum

SECOND STAGE

- When has exhausted his energies, his memory is full of his sexual achievements.
- Can have an orgasm without an erection by imagining a young girl.
- Great fear of suffering—have seen a lot of suffering.
- Very brusque in interview initially—in a hurry—may prescribe Nux initially (or Sulph.). Anxiety does not reveal until later.
- When they are suffering they tolerate it quite well, but fear it will develop into something i.e. fear of suffering in the future.
- > cold applications, cold water, cold shower.
- < warm applications, warm drinks.
- Distorted nails.
- Hair sticks together and falls out.
- Epithelioma.
- Develop flabbiness, especially vascular system.
- Varicose veins.
- Prolapse rectum, uterus.
- Constipation—anxious about it.
- Very anxious about delayed menses—fear cancer.
- Prostrate hypertrophy—frequent urination.
- Headache if ignore desire to urinate.
- Frequent painful erections at night (Carcin, Staph).

SLEEP: Falls asleep immediately, wakes in 3-4 hours with sexual thoughts and erections. Sleepless for many years.

DIFFICULT TO TAKE CONTACT WITH
IRRESOLUTION
DEPRESSION FROM MUSIC
PHOTOPHOBIA

GRAPHITES NATURALIS (*graph.*)

The main idea which comes to mind in Graphites is BLANDNESS—a dullness and heaviness on three levels. It is as if these patients are "thick-skinned" or "calloused". They seem to have a barrier which prevents stimuli from the outside world from reaching them. Outside impressions do not seem to penetrate, resulting in a blandness of the entire systems.

In physical appearance, Graphites patients are generally overweight and flabby. They often have dark hair, and the skin colour tends to be earthy. The clinical appearance has many similarities to that seen in cushings disease. Graphites is not as flabby as Calcarea; indeed they may be labourers by occupations. The Graphites skin is not as white as in Calcarea; it has the appearance of greater vitality. As a general rule, Graphites pathology seems to effect most frequently labourers, villagers, truck drivers etc.

Graphites shows a lack of sensitivity to any stimulus—body, emotions, and intellect. Any type of intellectual, analytical, or scientific work is difficult for Graphites patients. The mind is dull, lethargic, show to receive information. The blandness of intellect comes about because only some impressions actually manage to get through to the patient's awareness. During the interview, this situation becomes apparent in the bahaviour of the patient. He provides few symptoms of his own volition, and he answers questions only superficially. To the interviewer, it seems difficult to make contact in any real way with the patient. It is as if there are callouses on his mind preventing anything from penetrating.

As one would expect from this insensibility, Graphites patients have a poor memory. Primarily this is a weakness of short-term memory—poor memory for 'recent events' as recorded in the books. The events of everyday life do not make a full impression on the intellect, so they are not clearly recalled. This does not, however, affect memory for events in the distent past prior to the onset of the Graphites mental pathology.

Eventually, the mind becomes empty. This is not quite the classic emptiness of mind seen in Phosphorus, which is more of an emptiness arising out of physical weakness. In Graphites, it is an emptiness of thinking itself. It is an absence of thoughts. They feel that nothing is happening inside. Sometimes this may also be described as a sensation of fullness inside the head which blunts the thinking. As with most polarities in Homoeopathy, either of these extremes can apply in Graphites.

Because of the dullness of mind, there is also irresolution. Graphites patients cannot make even the simplest decisions. They may go into a store and spend a lot of time trying to decide whether the price is good or not. Finally, because they cannot make up their mind, they leave the store empty handed.

Eventually Graphites patients become aware that their mind is not working properly. This awareness then leads to various anxieties. In particular, they develop the fear that something bad is going to happen. They are aware that they do not quite comprehend everything that is happening, so they feel a calamity is going to strike. This is not so much the fear of insanity that is so characterstic of Calcarea. Rather, it is a fear of some misfortune impinging upon them from the outside world.

All of these mental and emotional symptoms are worse in the morning—especially upon waking; the blandness of intellect, the anxieties, the fears, the irresolution, and physical sufferings as well. They do not want to do their work, especially if it involves intellectual effort. By evening, however, the pressures of the day let up, and they feel relieved. In the evening, they may be capable of becoming excitable—even emotionally aroused. Nevertheless, by the next morning, the pathological state again reappears.

Whenever Graphites patients are in an unhappy mood, listening to music makes them feel even more miserable. This is not like Natrum mur. patients, whose sensitivity is more refined—romantic and sentimental—and who indulge their depressions by listing to music. In Graphites, it is an actual aggravation. Music makes them feel miserable, and they cry out of self pity.

On the physical plane, the skin is the major focus of pathology. Just as we see thickening and sclerosis on deeper levels of the organism, there are thickenings in the skin. Graphites has a prominent tendency to form keloids after a wound or a surgical operation. I recall two cases which were greatly benefitted by Graphites on this indication.

Similarly the discharges in Graphites are thick and sticky. Just as the mind is thick, hardened, and difficult to penetrate, so are the skin and discharges.

Graphites, of course, is famous for all kinds of skin eruptions, especially the most severe types. There may be eczemas affecting the whole body, herpetic outbreaks, scaling eruptions, etc. The most frequent areas affected are the antecubital and popliteal fossae, around the margins of the scalp, and in the ears. There may be cracking of the affected areas (especially in the ears of children), and the discharge of yellowish, thick, sticky fluid—looking like serum—is offensive. These specific characteristics of the skin eruptions are highly characteristic of Graphites.

A related keynote of Graphites on the physical level is brittleness and deformities of the nails.

Graphites is one remedy which suffers greatly from any suppression of eruptions. If cortisone or other medication is used to suppress an eczema, the patient may well develop asthma, headaches, or duodenal ulcers. The stomach is often a particular target of pathology. There is cramping and burning in the stomach which is immediately and dramatically ameliorated by eating. This, of course, is a symptom found commonly in ulcer patients, and therefore cannot be considered a strong guiding symptom. Nevertheless, you will see it combined with the rest of the Graphites symptomatology. The patient feels a cramp in the stomach, and all he wants to do is lie down, keep quiet, and have something to eat.

A peculiar aspect of Graphites patients is that, although their complexion is generally earthy, they become flushed just before experiencing a physical symptom. The face flushes, and as the flush subsides, they have the stomach pain or the headache.

Photophobia is a strong characteristic of Graphites, as it is with the Natrums in general. The leading remedy having photophobia is Natrum sulph., but Graphites is comparable.

Another striking physical symptom is numbness of the extremities. Graphites is the leading remedy for this symptom in general. This may affect the arms, the hands, the feet, the fingers,

Graphites Naturalis

or the toes, but it most frequently involves the forearms. Generally, these numbnesses are associated with cramps. When the numbness affects the TIPS of the fingers, however, think of Phosphorus.

Graphites is generally left-sided, and it is sensitive to cold. In keeping with its general insensibility the sensitivity to cold does not seem to be so much of an intolerance to wet weather or to change of weather. Rather, it seems to be internal.

The food symptoms in Graphites are distinctive. Graphites has an aversion to salt, sweets, and fish. It is the only remedy which has this combination. In respect to salt and sweets, it is interesting to compare Arg.nit., which is just the opposite. Arg. nit. craves sweets and salt, and it is a high-energy excitable, warm-blooded remedy. Graphites, on the other hand, is a chilly, bland remedy with an aversion to these foods. In addition, Graphites has a strong desire for chicken.

As always, these keynotes must not be prescribed upon in themselves; they must always be fitted into the general picture—the lack of contact, the blandness, the general appearance.

When one considers the tiredness, the fatness, the coldness, the glandular affections, and the flushing, it would seem easy to confuse Graphites with Ferrum. However, in Graphites, the fears come mostly in the morning, and the dissatisfaction, irresolution, and fear that a calamity is going to occur help to differentiate Graphites. Pulsatilla can sometimes be confused with Graphites because the irresolution can appear to be a kind of changeability. Of course, Pulsatilla is warmblooded and is aggravated in the evening after twilight. Many cases present a dilemma between Graphites, Ferrum, and Pulsatilla. In these situations, the differentiating parameters are the effect of open air, how fast the patient wants to walk, and the food desires and aversions.

Another remedy similar to Graphites is Calcarea, of course. It is chilly, obese, and easily exhausted by mental work. Graphites has a definite aversion to mental work—an almost anti-intellectual condition. Calcarea, on the other hand, may suffer from mental exertion but will continue to perserve in an effort to complete the task. Also Graphites is more physically robust than Calcarea. Graphites patients may be more crude and coarse—

like villagers, for example—but they can do a lot of physical labour.

Correlating with the blandness of intellect in Graphites, it is interesting that such patients do not seem to degenerate into DEEP mental pathology. They may live to old age without any particular mental imbalance OTHER THAN THE BLANDNESS. It seems they do not suffer from the types of deep disturbances found in the modern, mentalised urban environment.

IRRITATION
NYMPHOMANIA

GRATIOLA OFFICINALIS (grat.)

- Female remedy, mostly affecting gastro-intestinal tract. Gastritis, duodenal ulcers, distension, rumbling.
- Nervous system; makes person nervously weak. Dissatisfaction, irritated (compare Cham, Nux). Depression of spirits. Tremendous sexual excitability, crave sex which does not satisfy. Nymphomania, then more tired.
- Left sided. Ovaritis, neuralgia, renal colic (may confuse with Platina).
- A sense of inefficiency—try to cover it up.
- Head feels small (opposite Platina—others become smaller).
- Local excitability of genitalia.
- Feeling of cold in abdomen and stomach.

HEPAR SULPHURIS CALCAREUM
(*hep.*)

To summarise Hepar sulph. in two words, one could say; OVER-SENSITIVE and ABUSIVE. Hepar patients appear as if their nerves are on edge, as if the nerve endings are raw and exposed. In this state, they feel as if they are going to break apart, that they cannot take the slightest pressure—whether physical or psychological. Then they become angry, nasty, vicious, and abusive of other people.

In the first stage of pathology in Hepar, there is a general weakness and sensitivity. They may become irritable over small things, but this is still controllable situation.

Next, there is a nervous excitement. Everything is done in a hurry. He speaks fast, eats fast, drinks fast, etc. The nervous system becomes would up into a super-excited state. This state of hastiness is most comparable to Sulphuric acid in its intensity.

As the nervous system pathology becomes more extreme, the over-sensitiveness becomes most evident. At first, this is manifest in the typical Hepar sensitivity to cold. Hepar is aggravated by dry cold air, especially by dry cold winds. Humid, cold weather, which bothers most people, is not so severe for Hepar patients.

A memorable peculiarity of Hepar is its sensitivity to cold surfaces., Touching such a surface with only the fingertips can bring on a general aggravation. Again, in this symptom we see the concept of exposed, oversensitive nerve endings. There is an IMMEDIATE reaction—a cough or a chill—without delay. Even sticking a hand or a foot out from under the covers may bring on these symptoms.

Hepar sulph. is aggravated by open air, any kind of draft, cold dry winds - all these are intolerable to Hepar patients and bring on generalised aggravations. This is why Hepar is considered one of the best remedies for progressed stages of the common cold. It is not wise to give such a deep acting remedy for an ordinary common cold. If you have given Aconite, Bryonia, Gelsemium, etc. but the cold has nevertheless imprinted itself deeply on the organism as a sinusitis or chronic bronchitis, especially when

Hepar Sulphuris Calcareum

cough is a prominent symptom, then Hepar may be considered. It should be considered a third level remedy for colds and flus.

Hepar patients have an INTOLERANCE TO SUFFERING in general. Whenever there is a physical ailment it manifests on the mental level as an intolerance to suffering or pressure of any kind. Their whole nervous system is in a fret. They become angry, nasty, abusive. They may not be able to find a real reason why they should fly into such anger. A woman is nasty to her husband over the smallest things, and she knows they are small things, yet she cannot control herself. A husband swears at his wife and children, seeming to blame them for his own condition. Hepar patients abuse other people because of their own intolerance to pressures, stresses, or suffering. They seem to hold other people responsible for their own problems.

Such patients fly all to pieces if they experience stress. For example, consider a Hepar woman whose husband is unable to bring any money home. She lives in a constant fret. She cannot sleep. She is anxious all the time over every little thing. When you take her case, however, it is difficult to find the remedy because she talks so rapidly and excitedly. She gives you a hundred tiny syptoms, but no clear picture. She pleads constantly with you to help her. Her suffering is "so great, you MUST help me! I am in so much pain, I cannot tolerate it any longer". You try to find modalities and characteristic symptoms, but all she does is complain and plead. Finally, what strikes you is that there is such great suffering over relatively minor CAUSES. Then your mind goes to Hepar.

The abusiveness, especilly verbal abuse, is the most characteristic situation for Hepar. You may encounter, however, a submissive woman who is completely dominated by her husband. Because she is forced to control her verbal expressions, her bodily sufferings are proportionately increased.

Another consequence of controlling the anger is the development of impulses to kill. A woman may have a strong desire to kill her child (like Sepia or Nux vomica) especially whenever she holds a sharp knife. I have never seen a patient actually carry out such an act, but the impulse can be quite strong. A small child, however, might actually stab someone while in such a state.

Another impulse I personally have seen in Hepar patients is the desire to set things on fire.

Finally, as the pathology progresses to a deeper state, a depression comes on. They think about the abuse, the swearing, and the destructive impulses, and they come to view themselves as full of serious weaknesses. This is when they begin to have suicidal thoughts. With Hepar, however, this is not a true suicidal wish—as it is in Aurum. This is merely suicidal thinking—more like Nitric acid. Of course, Hepar patients do not have the anxiety about health or fear of death seen in Nitric acid and other remedies. It is merely a dwelling on the idea of suicide.

On the physical level, there are a few peculiar symptoms. As mentioned, there is the generalised aggravation from touching a cold metal surface, or sticking a part of the body out of the covers; even the draft from an air-conditioner can create a general aggravation. Also, Hepar patients may have an inclination to weep just prior to coughing; this is not because of anticipation of the discomfort, but simply an inclination to weep. There are, of course, the splinter-like pains for which Hepar is famous, especially in the throat; this is a very prominent symptom in Hepar. Finally, Hepar has desire for acids, especially vinegar (not lemon).

Hepar is very famous for suppurations and long-standing discharges. This points up the similarity to Calc. sulph., which is the sulphate of calcium, whereas Hepar is the sulphide. How does one differentiate? Calc. sulph. and Hepar are both intolerant to cold, but Calc. sulph. is not as severely chilly as Hepar. Calc. sulph. is more aggravated by humid cold, rather than dry cold as is Hepar. In addition, Calc. sulph. is not as excitable as Hepar. Even with these points, however, the differentiation can often be quite difficult.

Nux vomica can be compared to Hepar. Both can be very irritable, violent, and abusive. Generally, however, Nux vomica is more self-controlled. Also Nux vomica patients do not complain so loudly over their sufferings.

Sepia can sometimes appear similar to Hepar, especially in the desire to kill her children. However, Sepia is not so nervous. Her mind is more dull. Sepia represents a condition of stalemate—a balancing of opposing forces. Hepar represents an imbalance—a "flying off the handle."

HYDROPHOBINUM LYSSINUM (*lyss.*)

Frist time used it had a very severe case :

- Rich lady, too sick to come to the office.
- Could not go further than her own block of houses, even in her Rolls Royce.
- Agoraphobia and claustrophobia.
- Eyes were glistening and wild and very vivid and fearful.
- Arrived perspiring—tremendous anxiety.
- Said for 15 years could not leave the house.
- If car stopped in front of hers—had a tremendous crisis and had to get out of the car and send someone to fetch it.
- Fear of something she swallows sticking in her throat, a piece of apple stuck there once.

Gave a series of remedies for one and a half years (at least 10 remedies) a little better but did not hold.

- Thinking fast. Very alert. All the senses heightened.
- When she became accustomed to coming, wanted to come once a week.
- *Then one day she said she left a tap running and immediately had to go and urinate.

Asked her if she had been bitten by a dog and had rabies vaccination. She said yes, age 5. R_x. HYDROPHOBINUM.

- Eruption broke out +++ shoulders, arms and back.
- Feeling of tongue filling the whole mouth to make her choke.
- Thoughts of suicide and doing something violent.
- Mental depression—feel stupid—unable to comprehend anything. Other times : mental AWARENESS AND EXCITEMENT.
- Quite forceful and abusive about others. Think people abuse them.
- Very critical and scolding.
- < seeing water, hearing running water.
- Fear of choking even without eating. Have to have a bottle of water with them all the time in case of choking. Have

to drink little sips when feel choked. May faint with anxiety if doesn't have water with her, though may never use it.
- Complain +++ that suffering hell.
- Fear of insanity—think it will actually happen to them.
- Fear of being alone—want someone next to them all the time.
- Impressionability.
- Emotionally cold and hard, but impressionable.
- Mentally quick, alert and aware.
- Glistening surfaces <.
- Great difficulty in swallowing big pills.

HYOSCYAMUS NIGER (*hyos.*)

This remedy is commonly thought of in the category of acute states, like Belladonna and Aconite, but it also has extremely wide usefulness in chronic conditions.

The mania in Hyos. has many similarities to that of the other remedies, but it is more passive in quality. The person is not as active, energetic, or violent. He is more pre-occupied with an internal state, sitting and muttering to himself, or talking to absent people, or to dead people. This is the kind of mania commonly seen in elderly senile patients—sitting alone, muttering about nonsense, picking at their clothes, oblivious to their surroundings. Of course, when pushed, Hyos. can explode into violence like any of the other remedies, thus explaining the fact that it is listed in bold type in the Repertory for Violent.

The basic disturbance in Hyos., in all of its stages, is jealousy and suspicion. Jealousy seems to motivate much of the behaviour, including the occasional violent outbursts. This may begin with jealousy over his wife, or the suspicion that everyone at his job is talking about him behind his back. This state then grows to include more and more people, widening the circle of suspicion from intimates and colleagues, to acquaintances, and eventually to complete strangers. The result may eventually be a simple paranoid state in a person who is still within contact with reality, or it may become a florid paranoid schizophrenia. It may even include some cases of delirium tremens, full of suspicion, imagining insects crawling all over him, seeing people outside the window who want to kill him. Such paranoids are common in mental institutions nowadays, afraid of everyone, convinced that people are trying to poison them, refusing food and medicine because it is poisoned.

There is also an obsessive character to the Hyos. mental process. Again, it is as if the defences of the organism, when confronted with the rising insanity, choose to compensate by causing the mind to become stuck in a rut, to become obsessive over simple and relatively harmless things. Kent's description is best on this:

"Hyoscyamus has another freak in this peculiar mental state. Perhaps there may be a queer kind of paper on the wall, and he lies and looks at it, and if he can possible turn the figures into rows he will keep busy at that day and night, and he wants a light there so he can put them into rows, and he goes to sleep and dreams about it, and wakes up and goes at it again; it is the same idea. Sometimes he will imagine the things are worms, are vermin, rats, cats, mice, and he is leading them like children lead around their toy wagons just like a child. The mind is working in this—no two alike; perhaps you may never see these identical things described, but you will see something like it that the mind is revelling in, strange and ridiculous things. One patient had a string of bedbugs going up a wall, and he had them tied with a string, and was irritated because he could not make the last one keep up." Such obsessive and picky ideas are commonly seen in delirium tremens, as well as in senility.

As the insanity progresses, it finally explodes into the sexual sphere, causing the erotic mania characteristic of Hyos. The person becomes shameless, exposes his or her genitals to anyone, plays with the genitals ceaselessly. There is manically increased sexual desire and behaviour. In speech, singing and cursing there is constant reference to sexual subjects. The other remedies also have lewd behaviour, speech and singing, but not so strikingly emphasised as in Hyoscyamus.

Here it is as if the unconscious, which was previously controlled by obsessive and paranoid ideation, finally erupts on the instinctual level and is there contained, without going on to the degree of violence seen in Stramonium. It seems to be true also that Hyos. acts most effectively in people who tend to live on the instinctual level in their normal life, governed by immediate needs and whims or impulses. It may also benefit people of a more spiritual nature who are obstructed or hung-up in relationship to the dilemma over sexuality and instincts.

The outbreak of the unconscious affecting the lower regions of the body also affects the functions of defaecation and urination. The person develops involuntary loss of stool and/or urine, during the day as well as at night. As in the senile dementia, the patient may spend hours playing with his stool, or merely sitting or lying in it without awareness. Such a symptom may even show up in a child without the rest of the symptomatology of Hyos. The child may develop involuntary urination for no reason; he is taken to doctor after doctor, many tests are performed, but the final conclusion is that it must be a psychological disturbance, since there is nothing physically wrong. Think of Hyos. in such a case.

Hyos. like Veratrum and Agaricus, has a great deal of twitching of muscles. It is also a remedy with wide action in convulsive disorders. There are many involuntary gestures, such as picking at bedclothes, picking at things in the air, etc.

The acute Hyos. delirium is characterised by much twitching of muscles and a passive mania. Hyos. has less violence and less intensity of fever than either Belladonna or Stramonium. The delirium may pass into a stuporous or comatose state. The patient may be roused up, give a reasonable answer to a question, then lapse back into stupor. Its acute stage also has hydrophobic symptoms; there is a dread of water, a fear of hearing running water, convulsions caused by hearing running water, involuntary loss of stool or urine upon hearing running water.

In comparison Hyos. is more passive, less violent, than the other remedies except in the extreme paroxysms or states. More than other remedies it focusses its activity on the sexual sphere, and on urine and defaecation functions. There is more jealousy and suspicion, and a particular kind of obsessive thinking over little things. It has twitchings like Veratrum and Agaricus and convulsions like Stramonium and Belladonna.

IGNATIA AMARA (*ign.*) (first version)

Ignatia is frequently indicated today, because of the women's liberation movement. Prescribed 10 to 15 times more for women than men. This woman wants to liberate, assert herself. Sensitivity coupled with romanticism. Ability quick, clever, artistic, women of today. Receptive, but deep down a kind of romanticism. That romanticism will eventually come into conflict with reality. Tries to assert herself, so that she would be equal to man. Sensitivity, romanticism, ability, frustration on any level in the world. She is imposing upon herself the logical conclusions, she will say I must do this, do that : she is capable of performing it. She can do things, so takes a lot of things upon herself, over—working taking on many more things than she could normally do. Becomes proud of herself, in the way she can handle situations. Irritability, changing of moods, sharp, fast, yet sensitive, deep down romantic. Overstrained, grief, vexation, a frustration in her job, and then there is a breakdown. In a breakdown, she will go into spasms, hysterical, unable to think or talk; pale, breathing deeply, a kind of hysterical collapse; like fainting. Will not respond to someone talking to her. At the moment of this shock, she is unable to cry. Later, she will go inside, lock the door and cry. A sobbing crying, goes almost into spasms. Conflict of romantic ideas with reality. Always has inside ideas that do not correspond to what the liberation movement requires. She goes through the shock, then she says,"What a silly thing I did,"she keeps on brooding. Will keep it to herself and not talk (Nat. mur, Phos. ac.). Silent grief. Will talk insanely, illogically, at the time of the grief. At that moment, she will not react to logical reasoning. Crowding of thoughts within. Trying to understand what is happening to her. If the shock passes, mostly the body is affected by cramping pains, neuralgias that have no pathological origin, but started from the time of grief and stress.

Physical problems may come on after feeling better on the emotional plane. They develop, in appearance, they lose their femininity. There is something hard about them. There is a slight hair growing on the face. After the shock she becomes hard, and indif-

Ignatia Amara

ferent to being liked by men any more—something cold and hard about her.

You must go slowly with them, because they get irritable and insult you. If you ask about emotional things, the patient may start to cry—she tries immediately to compose herself. She will be withdrawn immediately, reserved. If she can't control, it comes out as a hysterical crying. when she regains control she will appear as if nothing has happened. Feels crying is the worst thing to do. Will go somewhere to cry alone. Hysterical sobbing and crying. Similar in reserved, introverted respects to Nat. mur. who will overcome her shocks easier. Ignatia will defend herself more from contact. Sudden shock that produces a state when they remain speechless, no way to talk out or cry. This is seen when there is a death in the family, or the severance of a relationship. Ignatia is not an emotionally stable person. Changing of moods very frequently. Can sacrifice herself for her parents. She flies into anger on contrary opinion of them. (When death occurs, she remains speechless because of the guilt). Gets hurt easily in a relationship. As a result, she gets nasty, then gentle, then nasty, so the man gets tired of her. She then becomes overwhelmed by emotion, if an unpredictable element is in her nature; changeableness. In her grief, she will say unjust things, accuse unjustly, becuase she is under stress.

Physically an emptiness in the stomach, not better by eating. More of a cramp of the solar nerve than the stomach. Affects the vagus nerve on breathing. She wants to breathe deeply; sighing. Either the stomach cramps or the sighing. She wants to eat, but the pain is not relieved. Perfers to be inside and in a dark room. Good food feels heavy in her stomach. Heavy foods have the opposite effect, are better tolerated, worse by fruits; they make her feel heavy. (Aversion to fruits with aversion to eggs—think of Phos.). Cramp can go from peripheral nervous system to deeper and deeper levels. Obstruction of the elctrical flow of the nervous system. Children develop choera-like symptoms, because of the remarks of their school teachers. (That is enough to bring on chorea in an Ignatia patient). Not a natural hysteria. (Hysteria —punishment of self and others, once the desire and the ability to reach out are frustrated. Moschas, Valerian, Lil. tig.) Ignatia is not such a deep pathology. Cramps; pains or numbness, from one point downwards. Cough has element of hysteria, seems to excite more coughing. So strong that she does not have time to breathe in. Does not have time to drink anything. Sudden momentary paralysis of parts. Inflamed parts, red, swollen, not sensitive to pressure. Better swallowing solids; worse when empty, or liquids.

Symptoms start after severance of love affair or death. Hurt very easily, becomes withdrawn and sulks; at this point cannot tolerate any contradiction of those closest to her. When in a love affair, she will suppress, until one day it will come out in hysterical reaction, she will accuse the man of coldness, of not showing enough attention, Sensitive women in our society, forced to be aggressive. She will suffer from the liberation movement. Eventually withdraws inside, sulks, over-protection of herself, becomes critical. Once alone, overwhelmed with a sense of loneliness. Grief. She will want to go back to the relationship. (Many times you will get the same remedy with couples). (Causticum and Phosphorous inimical). Great sensitivity inside, really a perfectionist. Does not accept the reality; how could he leave? Constantly dissatisfied with their emotional life. Out of their grief comes the attitude life is not worth living. She will be thinking of committing suicide, but she will not do it, she is too logical (but will think about it a lot).

If the mental level is affected, during the shock, she may develop a type of delirium. Torticollis, if things go into the physical with great force. Choera, cramping, unexpected reactions, to external or internal stimuli. Always expect these unexpected reactions from the Ignatia patient. Unexpected in the emotions; you are nice to her and she turns out to be nasty. Unexpected in the mental plane. Always an unpredictable manner in which she reacts. Can develop a hardness, criticalness, indifference to sex, not an aversion.

Homosexuality—(Sepia, Pulsatilla, Platina, Medorrhinum).

IGNATIA AMARA (*ign.*) (second version)

This remedy is frequently prescribed because of a technological civilisation. Woman 15 to 1 ratio to men needing this remedy. Sulphur will many times follow Ignatia—it lies underneath. Apis, Nat. mur, Sepia are complementary to Ignatia. A Nat. mur. patient after a shock or grief, may get prescribed Ignatia if you were to see them right after the shock; whereas if you had seen them before the shock you would have given them Nat. mur. Give the remedy that corresponds mostly to an uppermost pattern.

Ignatia individuals are very sensitive. An individual that has been brought up with culture, refind education, arts, music, theatre, becomes refined with culture. This parameter is coupled with the capacity of Ignatia to grasp quickly and execute quickly. Capable people. When these individuals are put in our society, their refined emotions can easily be hurt or disturbed. Become involved in the liberation movement, but it is not in their nature to be hard and cruel. This combination of factors will produce an Ignatia patient. At the same time she is capable, demands nothing from others.

Such an individual encounters a time, say about age 18 or 19 when she has been over working, and meets with her first love affair. She will believe in him totally. If the man at some time shows a little indifference, if she does not have total attention, she may become silent and brooding. The introversion may begin. This great sensitivity is the whole cause of trouble later on. She will withhold and not talk. Ignatia at a certain time may break down and become hysterical, make a scene of hysteria, out of control. From this point on we have pathology.

Wants to shout, but she sobs silently in her room. A lot of thinking going on in her mind. Feels she has been cheated in an affair, decides never to see him again. No humbleness in Ignatia. If she apologises for her outbreak, she is not calm about it. Tremendous indescribable anxiety, SIGHING. May sigh many times during the interview. When she apologises she means it logically, but not emotionally. Does not suffer much mentally; emotional level is the first one that suffers.

This shock seems to produce a cramp on the whole system, the emotions and the nervous system. May affect the vagus nerve. Unable to breathe properly sometimes, must take a deep breath. Ignatia may not cry. Will complain that they can't cry. (Cramping on the emotional level). Emotion is strong, but it is inside, cannot be expressed, unlike Phos. ac. where there is a paralysis of emotion with complete indifference. When she does cry, she will cry with sobs, so much so that the whole system will go into spasm. Instability, unpredictability, she says illogical things, insane things. Can't calm her down by talking to her logically. The same unpredictability will run through the physical symptoms e.g. eating the simplest food and can't digest, while eating heavy foods will feel OK. This shock in Ignatia can go deep enough to affect the hormonal system. If it goes deep enough, you may see traits of masculinity e.g. growing hair, or a kind of aloofness. Will sit back, take chair farthest away from the office. If she can't explain something logically, she becomes suspicious.

If such a state is left untreated for many years, she becomes more and more withdrawn into herself. A state of mind that can become diffused. A great irresolution, they can't decide. Also during that state is a fear of insanity. May develop anxiety about health. They feel they may die from heart disease or cancer. Anxiety worse at sunset, together with a sensation of constriction of the throat, i.e. hyperthyroidism where they feel a lump. Constriction in the throat. During such a disturbance she may stay in bed for several days because she feels something serious may come on. If married, she worries what may happen to her children if she dies. If progressed, may become the classical hysteria. Ignatia's hysteria-like condition may bring her down into spasm. Paroxysms of cough, in such order that you feel she may not have time to breathe. Cough is dry, appears sensitive, not much fever. Such states may exchange themselves for conditions like chorea. Especially in children.

After shock, goes on brooding, can't take a reprimand. Other layer may need to be eradicated under Ignatia in these choreas. Suppression of choreic movements builds up an energy that must be discharged at one time or another (or convulsions or distortions). Some elements of transient paralysis or a feeling of numbness. Something that is soothing for another patient may not help

Ignatia Amara

Ignatia. Nice clam words during a crisis will make her worse, like Nat mur.

Changeability in her character and in her moods. Jealous (Hyoscyamus, Lachesis). Lachesis will create in her mind a lot of stories about her husband being with a woman, all kinds of stories of what her husband is doing. Ignatia is the opposite, she will keep it to herself. She will not say a thing, will feel absolutely degraded to make a scene. In Hyoscyamus, it overtakes the person and paralyses them completely, as if somebody has caught them and is holding them there; indescribable feeling of jealousy, paralysis, constricted feeling in the cervical region. Nux vomica comes out in fits with great quarrels and irritability.

There is a state of Ignatia where everything is suppressed. She does not talk. May go into thoughts of suicide (mostly just the thinking may develop torticollis).

Keynote; aversion to fruits (all, kinds)—in 40% of Ignatia cases. Very few remedies have this (also Phos, Baryta carb.).

The Ignatia picture may develop after a death, separation of affair, marriage emtional disturbances.

KALI BICHROMICUM (*kali-bi.*)

Kali bich., like all the Kalis, is difficult to describe on the mental/emotional planes. All the Kalis (except Kali arsenicum, which is very similar to Arsenicm) are similar in personality; closed, reserved, able, rigid, and very proper. Kali bich. typifies this type of personality. NARROWNESS on all three levels is perhaps the most apt description.

Kali bich. people, by nature, are closed. They are people who are very conscientious and capable, and usually rather conservative. They tend to create their own little world, usually characterised by rigid routines, and they become quite content in the narrow context they create for themselves. They are set in their ways, and perhaps even unimaginative. A Kali bich. man, for instance, may join a particular political party in his younger years, and he dogmatically insists on the same point of view through out his life. He is narrow-minded and has difficulty seeing other points of view. In this sense, Kali bich. patients tend to be "squares".

Like most of the Kalis, Kali bich. patients can be quite materialistically-minded in their outlook. They enjoy their home, their family, their car etc. They eat well and enjoy food. They enjoy sex, and they insist on having it on a regular schedule. However, they accept traditional values; a Kali bich. patient is not likely to engage in adultery, for instance. They accept and insist upon the material point of view. Kali bich. patients would be the last to become spiritual seekers or mystics; and if such a patient does get involved in such a pursuit, it will most likely have a practical, scientific orientation.

Kali bich. patients are quite closed into their own world. They neither seek nor need company. They have emotions, of course, but they do not show them. A Kali bich. man feels perfectly content to stay alone, or only with his wife. He could be a literary man, focussed on his own paticular field, and content to remain so. He doesn't want any kind of interference. Even if someone comes to the door and rings the bell, he may not answer it.

Kali Bichromicum

The Kali bich. patient wants to spend time only with his family. He will be unlikely to have many friends outside the family, and whatever friend he may have he will welcome visits only infrequently. Taken to the extreme, then, Kali. bich. patients become misanthropic and antisocial. They close themselves into their narrow world.

Such a patient can be quite difficult during an interview. He will complain of a specific, concrete pain, and he will not want to go any deeper. If you probe intensively into the emotional or mental realms, he will deny any problems. You get the impression that he views such things as topics which are not to be discussed. At most, he may admit to a vague (and minor) irritability whenever he feels interference with his normal life.

There is, of course, a general weakness which affects all three levels of the person. On the physical level, it manifests as a general weakness, and as characteristic symptoms which will be discussed later. On the emotional level, there is easy discouragement and gloominess. Such patients always feel isolated and apart from social contact. When the Kali bich. pathology overtakes them, they do not share their feelings. Consequently, they become gloomy and ill-humoured. They become easily angered and upset.

Finally, this gloominess may progress into a kind of sullen indifference. This is not a true apathy in the sense we see in Phosphoric acid. It is more of a peevish withdrawal; a sullen indifference and discouragement.

Generally, the mental plane is not as definitely affected as in other remedies. Despite being emotionally closed and antisocial, they still perform their duties quite adequately. In cases in which the mental plane is affected, the first sign might be a weak memory. Next there may be some weakness in concentration, a blandness or dullness in the mind which duplicates the clouded feeling during sinusitis. Beyond that, I have not seen deeper deterioration on the mental level. It would not be difficult to imagine the result however; such a patient would most likely become psychotically withdrawn into an extreme misanthropic state.

There is a peculiar characteristic of the mental state which I have noticed in Kali bich. patients; because of their narrowness and lack of social contact, they seem to become excessively conscientious in explaining things to others. For instance, a Kali bich.

lawyer explains to you that you must bring this paper, this paper and that paper in order to sign a particular contract. To you this seems simple and self-evident, but he insists on making an elaborate, detailed listing of exactly why each paper is needed. In Kali bich. this is not a matter of orderliness or fastidiousness. It is a matter of going to an extreme to show you he is doing his job. He is trapped in his narrow, step-by-step, routinized way of thinking, and he naturally assumes that others think the same way. Therefore he takes excessive pains to explain every detail, even while you are impatiently wondering, "Why in the world is he doing this?" I have seen this narrow, arteriosclerotic kind of mentality in a man only 30 years old.

By far, the most prominent symptomatology in Kali bich. is on the physical level, which displays several highly characteristic symptoms. By following such cases over a period of years, I have found that there is an alternation of symptoms between the mucous membranes and the joints. At one point in time, you see catarrhs, then three, four, or six months later there are joint complaints.

When the joints are affected, the most typical characteristic is that the pains wander from joint to joint. One week, the pain affects one joint, and a week or a month later another joint becomes painful. Actually, the inflammation of the joint is truly another mucous membrane affection—involving the synovial membrane.

Characteristically, Kali bich. patients are ameliorated by warmth. Kali bich. patients in general are chilly, and their local pains are understandably ameliorated by warmth. It is interesting, however, that their complaints often originate during the summer. This is not an aggravation from heat, but a causation during the hot SEASON. By contrast, Pulasatilla has wandering pains, but is aggravated by heat itself; the heat of summer, but also the heat of a warm room, a stove etc.

Another famous keynote of Kali bich. is pains located in small spots —spots which can be covered by a finger. In my experience, the most characteristic location for such a painful spot is at the upper outer angles of the scapulae. just as Rhus tox. seems to gravitate toward the inner angle, Kali bich. seems to develop a trigger point on the outer angle.

Kali Bichromicum

The most well-known use of Kali bich. of course, is in catarrhal states of the mucous membranes. In Kali bich, it seems that once the pathological condition takes hold, it tends to progress more deeply. If such a person gets cold which is more frequently than usual, it progresses into a sinusitis in about 80% of cases. The progression may also reach into the Eustachian tubes, causing obstruction. There may be a considerable quantity of post-nasal discharge. Or, a cold may progress into a bronchitis or even asthma.

The most typical picture, however, is a patient who presents with sinusitis. You see a patient who has had frequent colds over the years, and every cold goes into the sinuses. A common cold starts, and suddenly there is a tremendous amount of discharge, the membrances of the sinuses swell up, the mind becomes dull, and the patient becomes despondent and even more peevish and anti-social than usual. Typically, the sinus pains most prominent are in the zygomatic region. The frontal sinuses seem to be less affected in Kali bich.

There is typically tremendous amounts of catarrh in such situations. The amount of discharge is profuse, and often it is characteristically ropy, elastic and viscid. The typical Kali bich. discharge, whether from nose, stomach, or elsewhere, is so stringy that it may stretch all the way to the floor. I have seen such a patient get tangled up in the discharge while trying to wipe his nose. Of course, mucous is normally somewhat viscid and a bit stringy. To be considered a symptom for prescribing purposes, however, it must be truly dramatic. Also, whenever this symptom is dramatic, it strongly suggests Kali bich. But its absence does not necessarily rule it out.

Even the most indolent ulcers which are found in Kali bich. display this symptom. You may see a patient who is quite closed, narrow in outlook, and arteriosclerotic to the point of developing a vascular ulcer which does not heal. When you try to clean it, you lift off the crust and observe several long elastic strings of serum attached to the crust. This observation, coupled with the general patient type, should bring to mind Kali bich.

As one imagine, arteriosclerosis is a major aspect of Kali bich., even at an early age. Such patients seem to narrow their lives —to sclerose their experiences, their emotions, and their attitudes.

Consequently, their arteries become sclerosed as well.

There are several characteristic peculiarities in Kali bich. One of the most famous, of course, is the sensation of a hair on the back of the tongue. In addition to this, the tongue is characteristically very shiny, rather than rough as usual.

Another characteristic of Kali bich. is its time aggravation, which is similar to Kali carb. Kali carb. is generally worse between 2 and 4 a.m. Kali bich. is aggravated in a narrow range, between 2 and 3 a.m.

The pains in Kali bich. can resemble Belladonna in that they come suddenly and go suddenly. In all other respects, however, there is no resemblance to Bell. Kali bich. patients are less strong, chilly, and anaemic-looking. The Kali bich. illness does not have the tremendous upheaval which is seen in Bell.

Kali bich. patients in general do not have particular food cravings or aversions, although they enjoy their food very much. There does tend to be a desire for beer, and Kali bich. is usually strongly aggravated by beer. This is not the usual distension and bloating which comes after drinking beer. In Kali bich, the whole person feels worse, the sinusitis or joint pains may flare up, or there may be diarrhoea.

Finally, whenever the Kali bich. patient describes a state of fear or anxiety, it seems to arise in the chest primarily. In Kali carb. by contrast, such feeling seems to originate in the solar plexus. In Kali bich., the root of the anxiety is higher. Also, there may be a deep sensation of coldness in the chest, especially a cold feeling in the heart.

KALI CARBONICUM (*kali-c.*)

As mentioned by Kent, Kali carb. is a remedy which is difficult to perceive in its essence both in the patient and in the Materia Medicas. The primary image of the patient is not readily available from provings, so it is known mostly by experienced homoeopaths possessing the skill of careful, systematic observation. It is very important to understand, however, because Kali carb. is a profoundly deep and long lasting remedy when prescribed early enough to prevent progression to an incurable stage of pathology.

The Kali carb. patient has a distinctive personality; committed dogmatically to strong sense of duty to an inflexible, rigid degree. It is an uptight state in which the mind maintains iron control over experience, behaviour, and emotions. Such a person is compelled to see the world in terms of black and white, right and wrong, proper and improper. In his appearance and behaviour he is correct, uptight, proper. He, or she, will be stoic, uncomplaining, dogmatic, by the book. In the field of psychology, the Kali carb. personality would be the epitome of the "anal-retentive" type. To such a person, life seems to be solid, clear, immutable, functional. Such people often become police officers, prosecuting attorneys, translators, bookkeepers—occupations in which routine, properness and the sense of duty are valued.

In this sense, the Kali carb. patient is overly mentalised. It is not mentalisation in the sense of philosophising or mental creativity or analysis, but rather an over-use of the mind as a mechanism for control over emotional expression as well as physical functioning. The Kali carb. mind is systematic, proper and routine-oriented. It thrives on clear-cut, black and white, dogmatic situations and functions.

Such a patient may appear to others to be devoid of emotions because emotions is expressed in a mentalised way, but this is far from the case. Internally, Kali carb. can be quite sensitive emotionally, but will never show it. If you tell a Kali carb. patient about your troubles, You will assume from his response that he couldn't care less, but you may be surprised to find a few days later that he has silently been dwelling on your situation and has come up with a solution. Such a patient, although suffering internally and silently, may be admired by others for dignity and integrity in the face of difficulties; the Kali carb. wife for example, may tolerate silently her husband's adulterous behaviour. On the other hand, a Kali carb. man can be frustrating to live with in a marriage, unless the wife is understanding enough to appreciate the indirect way in which such a person shows his feelings. He may appear to be devoid of emotions because of his controlled expression of them, but he may well feel things quite strongly (unlike, for example Phosphroic acid or Aurum met. which are internally truly dead and "still" in the emotional sphere).

It is for these reasons that the Kali carb. patient is difficult for the homoeopath to treat. Such a patient will stoically tend to ignore problems until they may have reached a serious stage. When he does come to the homoeopath, he answers questions with a matter-of-fact shrug of the shoulders. This is the patient who gives you no symptoms at all. You may ask if he has a fear of the dark, and the patient may shrug his shoulders in assent conveying to you a mild degree of intensity, whereas indeed the truth is that he is extremely afraid of the dark. The very symptoms which mean the most to the homoeopath, the emotional and mental symptoms, are the ones the Kali carb. patient downplays the most. This is a situation in which the homoeopath's skilled insistence of real life images and concrete examples, rather than mere recording of data can be crucial because the Kali carb. patient, left to his own devices, will allow his condition to reach an incurable stage before revealing the emotional intensity of his state. The toll that such mental control can take on the physical level can be illustrated by a sample case.

A Kali carb. wife was admitted by all her friends for never displaying self-pity or frustration while her husband slid into a troublesome senility over a period of many years before eventually dying; later, after suffering a financial loss, she developed a renal colic treated allopathically by an injection, and then rapidly collapsed into congestive heart failure and died.

Such iron-clad mental control prevents the final force from utilising its most important channels of expressions of symptoms on the mental and emotional levels. Therefore the symptoms become channeled with devastating force on the physical level,

Kali Carbonicum

especially affecting the internal vital organs, and the lower regions of the body. The mental suppression is so extreme, as a matter of fact that it seems to have a deforming effect on the structures of the body; it would almost seem that the extreme mental control distorts the structure of even the cells themselves. There are deformities of the bones, of the spine, and of the joints. (Kali carb. is almost a specific for deformative arthritis.)

The exaggerated mental control drives the symptoms expression most characteristically into the solar plexus. If he acknowledges emotion at all, he will describe it as being in the stomach—anxiety, fear, even shocks from the environment. Kent has a graphic description of this state. "A peculiar condition in *Kali carb.* is a state of anxiety felt in the stomach, as though it were a fear". One of the first patients I ever had expressed it in a better way than it is expressed in the books; she said "Doctor, somehow or other I don't have a fear like other people do. I feel it right here", (epigastric region). Well, that is striking, that is peculiar. It was not long before I developed another feature of *Kali carb.* By a little awkwardness on my part, my knee happened to hit the patient's foot as it projected a little over the edge of the bed, and the patient said. "Oh!" Sure enough, that was *Kali carb.* again, for you will find in Kali carb. a patient that is afraid and everything goes to the stomach, and when touched upon the skin there is an anxiety or fear or apprehensions felt in the region of the stomach." One patient I recall described a sensation of being struck in the solar plexus every time she would lie down for sleep; it was so severe that she was forced to get up and walk around in order to relieve the sensation. Another remedy having a striking similar sensation is *Mezereum;* it also feels a powerful anxiety in the stomach, but in *Mezereum* the anxiety arises from the stomach then overwhelms the whole organism, causing the person to feel as if he is dying.

So we see that the Kali carb. patient is quite sensitivie to emotions and to environemental changes, but maintains tight control over expressing this sensitivity. For this reason, we can also see the extreme sleeplessness present in Kali carb. Sleep is a time in which mental controls are naturally relaxed, something which is difficult for the Kali carb. patient. Such a person may go many weeks without sleeping, yet you cannot find any particular reason for the sleeplessness; the patinet denies anxiety, overactivity of the mind or sensitivity to noise. It is merely an unwillingness to let go. It may even seem that the patient, living such a highly routinised, systematic, proper life, seemingly deviod of stress, is in fact conserving his energy so effectively that sleep seems as if it would become unnecessary. However, the patient does suffer from the lack of sleep. Because he seldom gets enough sleep. *Kali carb.* is one of the remedies most strongly manifesting the symptoms. Unrefreshed sleep (along with, but for different reasons, Nux vomica, Lycopodium, Sulphur, Phosphorus, Nitric acid, the Magnesias, and Lachesis).

Characteristically, the symptoms of Kali carb, are aggravated between 2 a.m and 4 or 5 a.m. The sleeplessness , the cough , the cardiac dysphonea, are all worse at this time of morning. This is a time when the mental control mechanisms have their least force. As the control is relaxed, the symptomatic expressions become intensified—hence he wakes up with the characteristic 2 to 5 a.m. aggravations.

As the mental pathology progresses, the Kali carb. patient becomes very irritable. This again is an irritablity arising out of the sense of correctness, the sense of duty, the dogmatism. The Kali carb. patient has a defintie idea of what is "right", or the "right" way to do something, and will not tolerate deviation from that. It is an inflexible state of mind. In this way, he refuses to accept his illness; the symptoms seem to annoy him and then make him peevish and extremely irritable. The wife who is internally bothered by her husband's adulterous behaviour, will not attack him for that but will instead become angry with him over trifling things—something wrong in his way of going about his job, or his household functions. If a Kali carb. prosecuting attorney decides that the defandant is innocent, he will take the case to his superiors and will tolerate no excuses, of, say, political influences or the necessity to set a legal example; the Kali carb. patient would rather risk his career than compromise his sense of duty, even if this means carrying his inflexible stance to an irrational degree. (He would rather "fight than switch", as the cigarette commercial says.)

As the pathology progresses even further, we see the emergence to prominence of many fears and anxieties which previously played a minor, or unrecognised role in the patient's life. The

Kali Carbonicum

nature of the fears is representative of the Kali carb. inability to cope with uncertainty or potential loss of control. There may well be a fear of loss of control in certain social settings in which his social role is unfamiliar to him. There is a strong fear of the dark, a fear of the future, and a fear of impending disease. This is not a hypochondriacal anxiety about health so much as a fear of the uncertainties involved with a disease; disease is something which he cannot control himself. There is a fear of ghosts, of course, because they represent a non-solid realm, the existence of which he has previously strongly denied.

Unlike many other remedies, the stages of mental pathology in *Kali carb.* rarely progress all the way to insanity. Mental control in *Kali carb.* is not lost easily to such a degree. Instead the patient is liable to succumb from a deep illness of one of the vital organs. It is as if the mind has forced the pathology into the physical body with such intensity that the vital organs succumb before the mind degenerates to the point of insanity.

It is interesting that two of the main organs which suffer from the Kali carb. pathology are the primary organs of excretion of wastes—the kindneys and the lungs. It is as if the rigidity and inflexibility, the exaggerated sense of properness, has caused a distortion of the bronchial and glomerular membranes in an attempt to contain the toxins whose existence are not acceptable to the Kali carb. patient.

Inhibition of kidney function, of course, results in the well known dropsies of *Kali carb.* There are swellings around the eyes, of both the upper and lower eyelids. Most specifically, there are swellings, appearing like small bags, of the inner portion of the upper eyelids.

In the lungs we see a wide range of pathologies, from bronchitis to pneumonia and even tuberculosis. The cough is very violent, racking the whole body, incessant, with gagging and vomiting, and most aggravated 2—5 a.m. and by drafts.

Kali carb. can also affect the liver and heart in most extreme degrees of the failure, again most likely because the pathology has been allowed to progress too far before being properly acknowledged. This unrecognised progression into vital organs is described in Kent; "I can look back upon quite a number of cases of fatty degeneration of the heart in which I could have prevented all the trouble with *Kali carb.* if I had known the case better in the beginning. These cases are insidious, and indications calling for *Kali carb.* must be seen early or the patient will advance to an incurable condition. There is a breakdown and organic changes and you look back over these cases and say, if I had only seen in the beginning of this case what I see now it seems as if the patient ought to have been cured. We learn the beginnings of remedies as we learn the beginnings of sickness. It is a prudent thing for a homoeopathic physician to glance back over a case that he has failed on, or someone else has failed on, to study its beginnings and see what the manifestations were. This kind of study to the homoeopathic physician is as delightful as post mortems are to the old school."

There are quite severe and varied symptoms in the gastro-intestinal tract. There is great flatulence and alternating constipation and diarrhoea, but most striking are the severely painful haemorrhoids.

The Kali carb. patient is exquisitely sensitive to even the slightest of ddrafts. s. The patient is so sensitive to a draft, or even the normal movement of air through the house, that he may go from room to room trying to find the source of a barely perceptible draft of no consequence to others.

When confronted with a patient of such extreme properness and mental control that symptoms are difficult to come by, we may be led to the remedy by the very presence of this essence, requiring only corroboration by one of the other key symptoms known in Kali carb. the 2 to 5 a.m. aggravation, the extreme sensitivity to drafts, the swellings of the inner upper eyelids, the anxiety felt in the stomach, the pathological states of the vital organs, and also the strong desire for sweets.

The essential qualities of *Kali carb.* can be reminiscent of other remedies to which it is related. Of course, one cannot study *Kali carb.* without recalling *Nux vomica*. *Kali carb.* however, is different from *Nux vomica* in its essence. *Nux* is highly ambitious and impulsive, whereas *Kali carb.* is quite content to remain in his routine, only then becoming irritable because of his sense of correctness and not because of frustrated ambination as in *Nux vomica*. It is nevertheless common to see a patient, after responding nicely to *Kali carb.* progress into a *Nux Vomica* state. Another remedy that may follow *Kali carb.* is *Phosphorus*, particularly once the Kali carb. solidity has loosened up enough to enable the more etheric *Phosphorus* sensitivities and fears to manifest.

LACHESIS MUTA (*lach.*)

Main idea is overstimulation, which is constantly seeking an outlet for relief, like a pot that is boiling all the time; needs an outlet or will break down. Snake poison; initially the poison goes through the bloodstream, stimulates first, and then on to more specific areas. Primary target is circulation (from study of Materia Medicas you must get the preference of remedies for certain systems). People with idiopathic high blood pressure. Flushes of heat in different ages. Haemorrhages, particularly where the colour is quite dark. Headaches, varicose veins, haemorrhoids, and all kinds of heart ailments. Appearances of ulcers and eruptions—a pink appearance, cyanotic, purplish. Sensation of circulation. Sleep is difficult. Rhythm in the circulation or in the morning. Sleep-morning, these are aggravating times for Lachesis. Worse by heat, if suddenly heated up, which changes the circulation. Worse after entering shower or a very hot room. Worse before menses—as soon as menses starts there is a general amelioration of the patient. Often feel a choking sensation in the throat. Wake up in a panic as if the breath has stopped. Lachesis leads all remedies in the symptom, "wake up in a panic", worse by a suppression of discharges. Outlet can even be restricted by the clothes, especially around the neck, also chest and waist. Psychological restrictions on the patient will have the same kind of intolerance.

If asked to do something immediately by his wife, he will feel the pressure. Intelligent. Easy flow of ideas. Pathology can reach to schizophrenia, talks and talks, changes ideas. May quit first job because he feels restricted. Overstimulation on the sexual sphere. Excesses on the sexual plane. Can produce a lascivious person. Obscenity, lewdness, can exhibit these. One of the main remedies for masturbation (the overstimulation leads to this), like Staphysagria and Platina. Origeion—masturbation in young girls.

Also it will be useful for acute rheumatic fever. Where there are usually valvular troubles in the heart, Lachesis may correct that.

Snake remedies affect mostly the heart and the circulation. Some will suppress the sex impulses, will suffer from the suppression.

One case, Lachesis was given because of sex suppression—can be typical of Lachesis. Left-sided kidney colic. Alcoholism—circulation can be out of balance; Lachesis is useful here. May produce a normalisation in the craving for alcohol. Lachesis even helps in delirium tremens. Also considered in cases where narcotics are taken.

Worse lying on the left side, aggravates all ailments. May have palpitations, dyspnoea, feeling of fainting. Lachesis prefers the left side with centralisation around the heart—left to right. Intercostal neuralgia—left side—Spigelia, Nat mur, Bryonia. Acute conditions—left sidedness. Congestion of the head; kind of bluish appearance. Sensitive to touch on skin or any constricition of the skin; least touch is painful, but deep is not so bad, (Belladonna congestions are more red than purplish, and more right - sided.) Sometimes amelioration comes by hard pressure (Bell. also has this).

Emotions are quite strong; quite attached to people and objects. The attachment is strong, so we get pathological conditions of jealousy. Can degenerate into jealousy or into lasciviousness (overindulgence in sex). One of the great self-centred individuals (read Kent's description of this self-centredness). A false idea of loving oneself—the other person that is connected becomes an object. If fears that he may love this object of pleasure, then you get this jealousy. Suspicion; imagining, during the jealous phase. One of the main remedies for people who are very suspicious. If jealousy progresses to suspicion, then may progress even further to paranoia. They may think that their family is scheming to put them into an insane asylum. Can go into deep states of anxiety and depression, worrying about their health, especially the heart. PARANOIA—Hyos, Kali brom. Tarent, Stram, Plat, Ver, Alb. Anxiety about heart diseases—Lachesis is one of the main remedies. Clairvoyant beings, have intuitions. Depression worse in morning, may feel quite moved, in afternoon it is quite OK. Left untreated, may go into continuous depression. Fear of insanity, at a certain stage (also Manc, Cann, Ind, Calc. carb.)

May eventually go into insanity. Crisis is worse just before the menses. Impulsive, sporadic type insanity. It occurs in fits. Locquaciousness; talkativeness when there is a suppression of sex. Replacing what is missing in contact and communication with

Lachesis Muta

talking and talking. One of the main remedies for religious affections. (If you suppress, you must have an outlet). Talking, jumping from one subject to another; such a flow of ideas passing through the mind, can't pass fast enough through the mouth. Very critical; they can't tolerate the least criticism toward themselves.

Lachesis has another state—has great ideas; frustrated in earlier years. Will not follow through on this ambition to do great things. All this driving inwards leads to development of kidney stones and heart lesions. This Lachesis is introverted, sensitive, does not want to hurt anybody, will never let out their emotions. You get these people who will not talk. Must understand that this type of silent person is also a Lachesis.

Wine will aggravate his case. Good speaker, but a bad conversationalist. When they have reached a certain mental state, a delusion appears; they will feel the dead people (their presence) talk to them. They will give orders to do things. Also, another remedy like this is Anacardium. Feels someone is talking to him, but Anacardium gets double feeling, one tells him to do good, and the other to do bad. The Lachesis desires and aversions—likes oysters very much, desires farinaceous foods (cereals, grains, macaroni, potato, pasta).

LYCOPODIUM CLAVATUM (*lyc.*)

Lycopodium is one of the deepest and broadest acting remedies in the entire Materia Medica, potentially affecting all conditions know to mankind. Despite its wide application, however, there is a central thread which runs through the remedy and clarifies its highly interesting image.

The main theme in Lycopodium has to do with cowardice. Inside, Lycopodium patients are constantly contending with cowardice—moral, social and physical. They feel themselves to be weak and inadequate, incapable of fulfilling their responsibilities in life, and so they avoid responsibilities. Externally, however, the Lycopodium patient may present to the world an image of **capability'** extroverted friendliness, and courage, which can make the true image of the remedy difficult to perceive without skillful probing on the part of the homoeopath.

The central idea in which Lycopodium shows itself in early stages is in relationship to sex. The Lycopodium patient seeks situations in which the desire for sexual gratification can be satisfied without having to face the personal responsibilities which are implicit in such intimacy. It is commonly observed in such patients that there has been a long history of one night stands, in which the patient seeks satisfaction and then walks away without further responsibilities. If a sexual partner shows interest in marriage, the Lycopodium patient becomes fearful of the responsibilities and whether he will be able to fulfill them. Usually, he will leave before becoming "penned in" by the responsibilities of marriage, children, or even other forms of commitment in life.

This relationship to sex is a superficial one. Gratification is the primary motivation; he wants it quick, easy, effortless and without consequences. If such a patient meets a secretary who is by chance alone in an office, the first thought on his mind will be that this is a sexual opportunity, and he will likely **make** advances. Such patient may also visit prostitutes frequently, as this contact implies no responsibilities. It is not as if the Lycopodium patient's desire is so intense, as it is in Platina; the Lycopodium

Lycopodium Clavatum

constitution is too weak for such intensity, but when the desire does arise, the Lycopodium way of handling it is focussed on the superficial gratification of the moment and the avoidance of responsibility.

Once married, the Lycopodium man or woman may well experience sexual dysfunctions because of the fear of being unable to fulfill responsibilities of intimacy. The woman may be unable to have orgasm or the man may experience impotence in the form of either premature ejaculation or absence of erection. Internally, the Lycopodium patient feels a deep state of inadequacy and weakness and this is challenged most noticeably in the intimate marriage relationship. The Lycopodium patient, sensing this feeling of inadequacy, usually presents strong, courageous, competent image to the world, but his bluff is called when responsibility and performance are required, as in marriage. So, it is in the marriage situation where administration of Lycopodium can have some of the most gratifying results.

Such patients are in constant fear that others will discover the truth about their inner state of weakness. They are constantly worried about what others think of them. Because Lycopodium fits highly intelligent and intellectual people, it is found frequently in professions requiring public performance—priests, lawyers, schoolteachers, even politicians. A priest may feel perfectly well before giving a sermon, but upon reaching the pulpit and realising that so many eyes are are upon him, he may suddenly suffer gastritis pain or great anxiety. Such a person may be able to carry out the task properly, but very often the physical or emotional suffering will seriously interfere with functioning. Again, this situation is a manifestation of anxiety in the face of responsibility, and the patient may well attempt to escape from his profession, sometimes semming to use the physical illness as an excuse.

Lycopodium patients may go overboard in presenting a bluff to compensate for the inner feeling of inferiority. They may exaggerate their attainments, their capacities, the people they know. They may go so far as to tell outrageous lies which cannot be supported when the moment comes to produce results. This bloating of their ego is a compensation for the presumed state of weakness inside, and it is based upon a powerful need to receive admiration and respect from others in order to "prove" themselves.

Eventually, the Lycopodium patient may end up becoming a

loner, a spinster, or a celibate spiritual seeker. By attempting to avoid responsibility and gain a measure of control over the desire for instant gratification, the patient may decide to become celibate. This is a fragile state of celibacy, however, because the Lycopodium patient is now constantly obsessed even more strongly by sexual thoughts. After years of discipline, the most pious celibate may break down with surprising ease once an opportunity is presented, only to immediately return to the disciplined state later.

In the second stage of development of Lycopodium pathology, the external bluff becomes even more exaggerated. The patient becomes dictatorial and tyrannical with those around who can be controlled. Lycopodium patients may be timed and passive with co-workers on the job who are not under their control, but become despots at home. A mother may be sweet to her neighbours but tyrannical with her children. By exerting power over others, such people attempt to generate their sense of personal power, just as they previously attempted to bolster their sense of power by seeking the admiration of others through lies and exaggerations.

It is also in the second stage that the Lycopodium cowardice becomes more intense. At this stage, many fears become evident. Lycopodium can become terrified by almost anything—being alone, the dark, ghosts, even strange dogs. It is because of such fears that Lycopodium patients, while basically loners because of their fear of facing responsibility, are said to desire company, but in the next room. There is a great fear of suffering of any kind; thus the Lycopodium patient can become anxious about health to the point of hypochondriasis. The fear and anxieties affect mostly the gastrointestinal tract.

In the third stage, prolonged dissipation of energy either in the search for sexual gratification or in struggling with the attempt to control it through celibacy, finally results in a deterioration of the mental functions. This may begin initially as a confusion or poor memory in the morning, and gradually progresses to a more marked memory loss and intellectual weakness. Finally, the patient degenerates into a state of imbecility or senility. Such patients are likely to end up in rest homes at a relatively early stage.

Lycopodium Clavatum

On the physical level, the *Lycopodium* appearance is fairly distinctive. There is an emaciation of the face, neck and upper torso. The tissues seem to waste away in these regions, while an exess of fat may accumulate around the abdomen, the hips and lower limbs. The face tends to be excessively wrinkled, particularly in patterns reflecting the prolonged anxiety and concern Lycopodiums have over what others think of them. The hair may become gray at an early stage and the person may appear considerably older than his actual age. the flapping of the alae nasi (outer boundaries of the nostrils), which is described so frequently in the books, is rarely seen in actual practice, because it is mostly limited to acute illness involving dyspnoea (laboured breathing).

The primary region of action of Lycopodium centres on the genitals, the urinary tract, the gastrointestinal system and the liver. This includes such complaints as impotence, frigidity, nephritis, peptic ulcer, colitis, haemorrhoids and liver disorders. The gastrointestinal tract, in particular, represents the qualities seen throughout *Lycopodium*.

Just as there is a bloating of the ego presentation in compensation for the inner sense of weakness, there is also a bloating of the intestines in reaction to weak digestion. The patient is "full of wind" and suffers severely after eating. Also, just as there is an emphasis on superficial gratification in sex, the Lycopodium patient frequently seeks gratification of the palate by craving foods, according to their taste—especially sweets and oysters. This comparison extends even further; the Lycopodium patient feels empty and unsatisfied after coition, and suffers excessively after indulging in a meal based on gratification of taste. Lycopodium patients are constantly trying to control their desire for such indulgence.

The weakness of digestion is frequently a consequence of a liver ailment. *Lycopodium* is often indicated in liver dysfunctions and it is interesting to note that the liver is commonly associated with mental disturbances which fit the Lycopodium image.

Lycopodium can be compared with many remedies, of course. The anticipatory anxiety which causes such suffering during public functions in *Lycopodium* can be compared to *Gelsemium*; in *Lycopodium*, it refers more to the state of suffering which occurs during the actual task, while *Gelsemium* is indicated more for the anxiety and symptoms which occur hours and days prior to the task. *Silica* is a remedy which has a lack of self-confidence, but it suffers mostly from the inablility to cope with any circumstance, not only the social and moral responsibilities which concern Lycopodium. Calcarea can have many similarities to Lycopodium but does not have the characteristic cowardice. Natrum mur. is also a remedy which presents an outer image in compensation for an inner weakness, but the Natrum mur. inner state is one of emotional and sentimental vulnerability rather than the sense of inadequacy felt by Lycopodium.

MAGNESIA MURIATICA (*mag-m.*)

Magnesis muriatica patients are people who eventually develop a SOUR temperament. They have a kind of bitterness, but one which is not hard or thorny. It is a dissatisfaction which shows vividly in the sour, facial expression. In their dissatisfaction they appear as if they are always in some degrees of anguish.

Mag.mur. patients are very sensitive to any kind of confrontations, either involving themselves or other people. They are pacifists—always trying to make peace. It is not that they are cowardly; in war situations they may display lots of courage. Their vulnerability is a purely emotional sensitivity. They want others to be happy and satisfied, and they may go to excessive lengths to bring this about. They will suppress their own emotions for the sake of others—not as much as Staphisagria, but quite strongly nevertheless. If parents fight, the Mag. mur. child suffers tremendously and tries to bring about peace. If an adult of such type has suboridnates at work who quarrel, he will work himself into an anxiety state trying to find a way to resolve the conflict.

Mag.mur. patients also have a STRONG SENSE OF DUTY. They easily overload themselves with too many tasks, and then become very anxious when they find themselves unable to keep up. They become overwrought with nervous energy trying to meet the demands and then find themselves unable to sleep properly.

This sense of duty, together with the emotional sensitivity to others, eventually leads to great restlessness and fidgetiness. Over the years, this nervous restlessness leads to sleep difficulties. In some cases they cannot fall asleep until almost morning. Others fall immediately into a profoundly deep sleep—like a log, or like a dead person—only to awaken in 4 or 5 hours completely unrefreshed. In either case, the normal sleep cycle is disturbed, and these people suffer tremendously from it. They never quite catch up, but they keep trying to run on nervous energy until finally they break down into weeping (which ameliorates in Mag. mur.) hysterical fits, or irritability and depression.

If you picutre in your mind such people who are sensitive, pacifistic, and duty-bound, you can see easily how they become introverted and develop a sour temperament. In order to avoid being hurt, they close themselvs off. But what distinguishes Mag.mur. patients is that they display this outward appearance of sourness, of dissatisfaction. They appear as if they are always in anguish, on edge, as if they can't take much more. They are completely unable to relax under any circumstances.

Mag.mur. is one of the leading remedies for unrefreshed sleep. This may be caused by subconscious anxiety, as mentioned, or it may be due to liver dysfunction. It is well-known, of course, that Mag.mur. is one of the remedies which are almost specific for liver troubles. Whenever the liver fails to function properly, toxins build up in the bloodstream and the patient wakes up in the morning feeling miserable all over. This is not the kind of morning aggravation seen in *Rhus tox*, which specifically affects the joints, which have been motionless during sleep. Rather, Mag.mur. patients awake feeling miserable in their entire being—mentally dull and unable to concentrate on their work, emotionally lifeless, and physically heavy and toxic (especially in the head). They describe this state as a **lethargy**, a feeling as if they had been drugged. It may take them a half hour to become alive, and then they become "overwound" until bedtime.

Mag.mur. offers us a golden opportunity to study the physiological effects of liver failure. It is interesting that in general people who are sensitive to conflict and develop a "sour" out-look on life, tend to develop pathology, with the liver as the target organ.

A primary characteristic of *Mag. mur.* is the aggravation from lying down—especially upon closing the eyes. The patient may feel relatively well until he lies down and closes his eyes to go to sleep. Then, all of a sudden, the restlessness comes on. He tosses and turns but is unable to get comfortable. Finally, he gets up and walks around a while. This relieves him, and he is able to go back to bed.

This aggravation from lying down applies to all symptoms in Mag. mur—the anxiety, the sleeplessness, and the physical symptoms. This can be a primary keynote during an acute ailment such as influenza. Because Mag. mur. is chilly, anxious, and restless, one might think of such remedies as Rhus tox or Arsenicum. Or, because it has the burning in the nostrils, one might

Magnesia Muriatica

consider Kali iodatum, Kali bichromicum, Arsenicum, or Allium cepa. However, the marked aggravation from lying down, and amelioration from being up and about, will lead you to *Mag.mur*. The patient may have a nasal catarrh which is tolerable under ordinary circumstances, but the moment he lies down and closes his eyes he starts coughing and choking severely. He is forced to get up, and then he is immediately relieved. This is exactly the opposite of Manganum, which is markedly relieved by lying down.

Another primary characteristic of Mag. mur. is the aggravation from salt. This probably explains why Mag. mur. is aggravated by swimming in the sea. The salt element has an adverse effect on the metabolism of these patients in general. After swimming in the sea, they not only feel worse in their local symptoms, but they feel completely drained of energy in general.

Mag. mur. is intolerant to cold in general. In spite of this, they may have warm feet—even to the extent of sticking them out of the covers. It belongs to a small group of remedies which are chilly but which also stick their feet out; Chamomilla, Phosphorus, Sanicula (Medorrhinum also sticks its feet out but is not so chilly).

Mag. mur. is chilly but also feels better in open air. It is also better from motion. Like Rhus tox., Mag.mur. patients will bundle up well and go out for a walk in the open air. This can be difficult to differentiate from *Rhus tox.* in some cases. The nature of the morning aggravation can be a keypoint, as mentioned. It would be very rare to find a Mag.mur. patient who is not aggravated in his whole being in the morning. Also, Rhus tox. has a strong desire for milk. *Mag.mur*. may have a desire for milk as well, but it is strongly aggravated by it. Milk causes a general aggravation and also a diarrhoea—mushy, unformed stools.

Mag.mur. patients often have a desire for sweets, and also for fruits and they have a strong desire for vegetables. Mag. carb., by contrast has an aversion to vegetables, especially to artichokes.

A few more symptoms which stand out in my experience; Mag.mur. prefers to sleep on the left side, and it is aggravated by lying on the right side. There are severe jerkings or electric-like sensations—especially when lying down. All magnesias are very sensitive to slight touch; *Mag.mur.* and Mag.phos. in particular are also better from hard pressure. There may be numbness of the extremities during excitement—such as during a crisis or irritability or hysteria.

I cannot say much about *Mag.carb.* since I have not yet gathered enough experience with it to understand its essence. From the experience I do have I can say that Mag. carb. patients tend to be more reserved right from the outset than Mag. mur. Neuralgias are quite distinctive, especially on the left side. It seems to diminish all five of the senses; loss of smell, loss of taste, etc. As mentioned, Mag.carb. has an aversion to vegetables. It also affects the liver. In my experience Mag. carb. seems to be more indicated than Mag. mur. in children who fail to thrive becuase of liver problems, especially if they have chalky white or yellowish stools. Mag. carb. children have the specific kind of weakness which prevents them from holding up their head. It is a remedy which even Kent seemed not to fully understand; he tended to use it as a last resort when other remedies ailed altogether.

MEDORRHINUM (*med.*)

Medhorrhinum is a remedy that goes to extremes in its pathology on all three levels. It seems incapable of maintaining a neutral, stable state. It is FITFUL, UNSTABLE, going from one extreme of pathology to the other. At one extreme, the Medorrhinum patient is highly sensitized; he or she seeks relief from sensitivity, and the relief is found in a state of PROFUSION. Everything is taken to excess—physical discharges, temper, impulses, sexual indulgence, etc. At the other extreme it is a state of INVERSION, a turning inward of the pathology to the point of suppression, timidity, and loss of physical, emotional, and mental power.

On the mental/emotional level, the Medorrhinum state of excess is almost maniacal—aggressive, forceful, wild. The nervous system and emotions become over-excited. Viewing this condition alone, one might think of such remedies as Tarentula or Nux vomica (although Medorrhinum doesn't go to such an extreme as Stramonium).

The same tendency is seen on the sexual sphere. A large part of the expression of Medorrhinum pathology centres on the genitals. The Medorrhinum man always thinks about sex, desires sex, when in the impulsive, aggressive phase.

His externalised aspect of *Medorrhinum* is one extreme. The other extreme results from a turning inward of all this energy. It becomes bound up and unavailable. The patient begins to lose power on mental, emotional, and physical levels. There is emaciation and atrophy—eventually even marasmus. The effects of suppression on any level are most evident by this process of inversion.

In this collapsed state the Medorrhinum patient experiences a loss of mental power. He is weak and confused. There is forgetfulness and absent-mindedness of all kinds—cannot remember words, cannot remember where something was left. Eventually, this progresses to a true confusion of ideas. Whereas before the mind was profusely expressive, now it becomes dulled, unclear, lacking in perceptive power.

Emotionally, instead of remaining in the externalised, wild state, the energies turn inward and create a state of over-sensitivity, reservation, and timidity. This is a state in such stark contrast to the other extreme that it is sometimes difficult to believe that one is seeing the same patient.

On the physical level, the externalised phase of *Medorrhinum* is characterised by an extreme profusion of dischares from all mocous membranes—conjunctival, pharyngeal, urethral, vaginal. We do not have an immediately visible opposite extreme regarding discharges, the pathology manifests instead as easy suppression of discharges into more deeply serious ailments. *Medorrhinum* discharges, when suppressed by allopathic treatment, for example, result in degeneration of deeper organs or further into the mental/emotional spheres.

As mentioned, the extremes of Medorrhinum pathology may manifest fitfully within the same individual. It is also possible to see these extremes as the dominant states in entirely different individuals; one aggressive and effusive, another timid and reserved—and both may require Medorrhinum.

It is rare in our Materia Medica to find a remedy manifesting such great contrasts. A keypoint to remember in *Medorrhinum*, however, is that both extremes are extremes in a PATHOLOGICAL degree, is not a situation in which there are paroxysms of symptoms and then a return to relative normality. When the pendulum swings in Medorrhinum, it goes to the complete opposite extreme of pathology.

For example, you may see one patient who is very fond of animals; if this is a Medorrhinum condition, the fondness will be carried to an extreme degree. The pet becomes the central focus of the patient's life, consuming incredible attention and energy, and perhaps even interfering with the patient's occupation. Another Medorrhinum patient may be the exact opposite. He may display great cruelty towards animals; he ties up his dog and beats it savagely over a minor annoyance. This is a true cruelty; while in this state the patient actually enjoys inflicting pain on animals. Later, however, the pendulum swings back again, and the patient goes into a state of excessive remorse. (Aversion to cats, can't stand cats, have a real fear of cats. There is an underlying tubercular miasm.)

Medorrhinum

They are very sensitive to beauty, to nice things. One type of Medorrhinum patient may be very deeply moved by the sight of flowers. This is not merely the healthy, casual, aesthetic appreciation of flowers that a young girl may feel on her way to school. This becomes an excessive emotional state—flowers become everything to the patient; she would be late to school and takes risks to steal the flowers! On the other hand, Medorrhinum individuals may be totally unmoved by the sight of flowers. This is not merely a lack of appreciation, it is an absolute disinterest in the entire realm of beauty.

The fitfulness of Medorrhinum is clearly seen in the fluctuations of energy experienced by such patients. They work very well for a short period of time, but then they collapse. They take on a project that requires a limited amount of energy, they work energetically and efficiently for two days, and then they are totally INCAPABLE of doing anything on the third day. If a project requires sustained effort over a long time, the Medorrhinum patient will most likely refuse to take it on.

The mental and emotional planes in Medorrhinum are closely intertwined. Nevertheless, it is possible to distinguish stages in the development of pathology. At first, there is forgetfulness and confusion on the mental PLANE. This confusion is similar to that of Alumina—an inability to understand or clearly express what is happening inside. The mental functions gradually diminish further, until it becomes evident that the patient may be sliding toward insanity.

At this point, we begin to see the peculiar fears of Medorrhinum. It does, of course, have fear of insanity. However, a specific fear that is most characteristic is the fear that someone is following behind him. The patient may be walking down the street and suddenly feels as if someone is behind him. He stops and looks but no-one is there. He cannot shake the impression, however; it sticks in his mind as a kind of "fixed idea".

Next, the mind develops a kind of internal wildness. There is the sensation as if a storm were occurring inside the mind. It is a wild, scattered, out-of-control feeling that is felt INSIDE. It is similar to the felling of hurriedness coupled with anxiety that we see in Tarentula, but it is more fitful. It is as if the clutch of a car had been disengaged suddenly, and the engine is racing out of control. As a consequence, there is a distortion of time sense similar to that in Alumina—time passes too slowly.

When severe enough, this stormy feeling reaches the point in which the patient begins to lose contact with reality. He or she feels as if everything is occurring in a dream. The mind becomes even more confused, unfocussed, scattered. Considering the sequence of development of symptoms, one could conjecture that *Medorrhinum* would be very useful in drug addicts who have broken down into disorientation in space and time.

The internal wildness of Medorrhinum is not apparent to an external observer. It is something which comes out when the patient tries to describe what is happening. The mind is internally disorientated and wound up, but not in the manner we see in *Lachesis*, for example. Lachesis can be very hyperactive but they can always think of five different words to describe the same thing. In Medorrhinum (and Alumina) there is great difficulty describing the sensation; it is as if the words were hidden behind a veil. The patient struggles for a long time and finally can only find the word "wild".

To the external observer, the appearance of an inverted *Medorrhinum* may resemble *Phosphoric acid*. He wants to say something but cannot. It is only upon further case taking that the full picture comes out. Phosphoric acid's "flatness" is continuous, not fitful as it is in Medorrhinum.

A prominent characteristic of Medorrhinum is relief with the onset of discharges. The patient feels quite well in mind and energy during a leucorrhoea, post-nasal drainage, or even a urethral discharge. If these discharges become suppressed, however, a deep effect on the organism is likely to ensue. There may be wasting, loss of tone of skin and muscles, and decline in energy and mental/emotional function. In addition's warts often appear after the suppression of discharges in Medorrhinum.

The effect of suppression does not affect the patient alone; it can be passed to subsequent generations as well. In this way, *Medorrhinum* is frequently indicated in marasmic children born of parents who are both strongly affected by the Sycosis miasm. These infants or children fail to thrive. They have very fine skin with an unhealthy white colour. They have no appetite at all, and eventually they suffer from malnutrition.

Medorrhinum

There are several symptoms which characterise *Medorrhinum* on the physical level. There are many rheumatic and arthritic sufferings. Particularly, in Medorrhinum patients suffering from rheumatic complaints, there is often great sensitivity of the soles of the feet; they are so tender that the patient cannot walk.

When discharges are suppressed in Medorrhinum, the direction is quite characteristic. First the mucous membranes are affected, then the joints, and finally the heart (considering, of course, only the physical level; deeper emotional and mental changes may occur concomitantly). Along with Lycopodium and Ledum, Medorrhinum is one of the remedies to recall in heart conditions arising after a streptococcal infection or rheumatoid arthritis. In addition, allow me to pass on to you a special precaution. When giving *Medorrhinum* to patients with significant heart pathology, or to patients above the functional age of 60 or so, do not give the initial dose in higher than 200 potency; this caution comes out of a few very unfortunate experiences.

Medorrhinum symptoms are characteristically ameliorated in the evening after the onset of darkness. This applies to symptoms on all three levels. This type of patient will very likely report to you, "I am definitely a night person. Don't ask me to do any real work during the daytime".

Of course, Medorrhinum is famous for its amelioration in the sea; this again applies to all there levels of the organism. In regions near tolerable swimming areas, this can be a very useful guiding NESS of the sea—as we see in Pulsatilla. In the repertory Medorrhinum is listed in several rubrics for food aversions and desires. In my experience, the most useful guiding sysmptoms here are desire for oranges and orange juice.

Medorrhinum in its essence presents us with an excellent example of the need for deep and careful case-taking and analysis. In different aspects, *Medorrhinum* can easily be confused with many other remedies. For example, the mental state can appear almost identical to Alumina—especially when you only see the patient in the office, separate from life stinuli. You must learn to VISUALISE the person in his or her life. Every patient appears as a saint during a medical consultation. Therefore, you must learn to pick up on every little hint. Stimulated perhaps by a glimmer in the eye or an inflection in the voice, you probe further for more descriptions, for living examples etc.

Eventually the patient may admit that there have been some occasions when he lost his temper and struck other people or animals. It is only after probing, however, that one can bring out a clear image of *Medorrhinum*.

Take as an example Nux vomica. It has aggressiveness, impulsiveness, and cruelty which could conceivably appear like Medorrhinum in its externalised phase. In Nux vomica, however, this is usually a very controlled state. It is controlled anger. When there is cruelty, Nux vomica has a CALCULATED maliciousness which is not typical of Medorrhinum.

Tarentula is a remedy which has the same hurried state. This is an overexcitation of the central nervous system which can be controlled by the patient. In Tarentula, however, it is a continuous state which finally leads to collapse. In Medorrhinum, the course of development is much more fitful.

These active remedies can be differentiated easily from medorrhinum by the fact that Medorrhinum goes to the opposite extreme of pathology. Medorrhinum becomes reserved, timid. In this respect, it is somewhat like *Thuja*. Both misrepresent themselves to other—they want to portray themselves as different than they really are.

EXTRA NOTES

Sense of hurriedness inside. They rush around saying "I have to do this! I have to do that!", but when they do something they are not methodical, systematic.

Desire for drinking. Desire for salt, sweets and fat; with a combination of these three think of Medorrhinum. (Desire for cheese—main remedies are Puls., Cist. can., Ignatia. Hyst.).

Children develop red, burning eruptions around the perineum, look red and fiery and make child complain all the time.

Sycotic remedies are better with humidity. With *Medorrhinum*, if they just sit next to the sea, they will be better.

Compare Syphilinum, much more slow and insidious. Different in their destructiveness. Medorrhinum is fitful, aggressive and momentary. *Syphilinum* has perversions in sex also; comes from a deep miasmatic cause, from generation to generation; starting at a very young age (i.e. homosexual), whereas Medorrhinum can come later on because of all his sex interest. Syphilinum is born as, Medorrhinum becomes as. Medorrhinum could commit murder in fits of passion.

MERCURIUS SOLUBILIS (*merc.*)

Study of *Mercurius* is a prime example of how the concept of the essence of a remedy can clear up a seemingly overwhelming mass of data. *Mercurius* being one of the more extensively proven and widely used remedies in the Materia Medica, presents a formidable array of symptoms for the beginner to study; it is a veritable textbook of pathological states. However, after repeated and prolonged study and meditation on the Materia Medica, one gradually is able to discern a thread, a theme, which runs through the remedy. Once this is comprehended, all the "data" falls in place into a single unique image.

In *Mercurius*, there is no single word or phrase which adequately describes this thread. The basic idea is that there is a lack of reactive power coupled with an instability or inefficiency of function. The healthy organism has a defence mechanism, a reactivity, which enables it to create a stable, efficient equilibrium upon exposure to the many physical and emotional stimuli in the environment. In Mercurius, this reactive power is weakened, becoming unstable and wavering in its functions. Virtually all stimuli are absorbed by the patient without adequate defence, resulting in a pathological condition.

The lack of defensive power results in the Mercurius patient being sensitive to everything. As we go through the Materia Medica we find that the Mercurius patient is AGGRAVATED by everything—heat, cold, outdoors, wet weather, change of weather, warmth of bed, perspiration, exertions, various foods etc. By contrast, there seem to be very few ameliorations; very little can be absorbed by the patient to result in comfort, because the system is unable to properly adjust to anything. As an interesting demonstration (though not a generally recommended method for study) one can go through the Generalities section of the Repertory seeking the number of rubrics in which it is listed in italics or bold type as being aggravated or ameliorated by physical influences; there are only 7 listings for amelioration (5 of which have to do with lying down), while there are 55 rubrics describing aggravations. Because of this extreme vulnerability, we see that the

Mercurius patient has a narrow range of tolerance to everything; for example, such a patient will be comfortable between only a very narrow range of temperatures, becoming uncomfortable from even slight heat or cold.

The intolerance to heat and cold illustrates the instability which characterises the particular *Mercurius* weakness. As mentioned by Kent, the patient is a living "thermometer". At one moment, he is suffering from cold and seeks warmth, but once warm he becomes aggravated by the warmth also. This is true not only during a fever, but also chronically. There is also a weakness and instability in emotional expression; weeping alternating with laughing. Unlike Ignatia, in which this symptom is a manifestation of a hysterical state from uncontrolled emotion, the Mercurius weeping/laughing is more of a mechanical instability. Once weeping, Mercurius feels a kind of mood come upon her which results in a swing to the opposite extreme of laughing; mechanically, laughing and weeping can often be quite similar, and so the *Mercurius* instability causes the patient to waver from one state to the other quite readily.

The Mercurius instability, its inefficiency in function, can be illustrated nicely by reflecting on the physical state of *Mercury*. If you break a Mercury thermometer, you discover that Mercury seems to exist in a state somewhere between a liquid and a solid. It flows like a liquid, yet it tends to retain its own shape to some extent like a solid. If you try to pick it up with your fingers, it seems to elude you; it does not allow itself to be grasped like a solid, and it does not stick to your skin like a liquid. In its physical form, *Mercurius* is erratic in function, just as it is unstable and inefficient in its pathological state.

Thus we can see readily that the *Mercurius* weakness is not like that of other remedies. *Arsenicum* can exhibit a prostrating kind of weakness, but it is quite unlike the instability of *Mercurius*.

Arsenicum, of course, shares many similar specific pathological symptoms, but the Arsenicum patient's cold intolerance is relieved by warmth; it is also true, of course, that mentally Arsenicum shows much more reactive power—anxiety, restless activity of mind, a shrewdness. *Stannum, Helonias,* and *Baptisia* are other remedies with severe weakness of reactive power, but not with the instability and inefficiency of *Mercurius*.

Mercurius Solubilis

This *Mercurius* weakness of reaction is not a sudden event. It is a slow, insidious process which can be difficult for the patient, and therefore for the homoeopath, to perceive in the early stages. It creeps up in such a slow way that the patient barely notices the vulnerability to stimuli. By the time the patient consults a homoeopath for a particular complaint the vast bulk of the symptoms have been forgotten, no longer being recognised as abnormal. Having learned to adapt to the narrow range of tolerance to things, the patient reports only the immediate symptoms which bring him to the consultation. In early stages, it takes patient, skillful and thoughtful questioning to elicit homoeopathic symptoms which the patient himself may not be aware are different from the experience of other people.

Because the mental state is the centre of being of the person, let us describe in detail the stages of development of pathology on the mental plane. The first effect noticed is the slowness of action of the Mercurius mind. The patient is slow to answer questions (like *Phosphorus* and *Phosphoric acid*, as well as other remedies). He is slow to comprehend what is happening, or what is being asked of him. This is at first not a confusion of mind, or poor memory, but an actual slowness, an incomprehension, a kind of stupidity. *Calc. carb.*, of course, also has a slowness of mind, but Calcarea is an intelligent person; once comprehended, *Calcarea* is able to use the idea efficiently. Mercurius is both slow of mind and poor in comprehension.

The Mercurius mentality has a kind of inefficiency in action. Mercurius is one of the remedies characterised by hurriedness and restlessness, but it is a hurry in which the person does not accomplish anything. A task which should take half an hour to accomplish will take the Mercurius patient one and a half hours. Remedies such as Tarentula, Sulphuric acid, Nux vomica, and Natrum mur. are also in a hurry to a pathological degree, but their activities are nevertheless productive and efficient.

The second stage is characterised by impulsivity. The Mercurius mind, because of the vulnerability to stimuli from without and from within, is unable to keep his mind concentrated purely in a particular direction. The healthy person is able to focus the mind on a subject or task despite the many random thoughts and ideas which may attempt to intrude. The Mercurius mind does not have the strength for such concentration. Every random thought which pops into the mind becomes something to which the patient feels a need to respond. This is related to the inefficiency of mind, but becomes even more extreme as the pathology progresses. Eventually the Mercurius patient becomes susceptible to every conceivable kind of impulse. He may have an impulse to strike, to smash things, to kill someone over a merely slight offence, or even to kill a loved one. (*Mercurius*, *Nux vomica* and *Platina* are the only remedies listed for this impulse).

These impulses, however, are not readily evident to the questioner. The Mercurius patient feels the urges, but controls them. He is a closed individual, slow to answer, reluctant to reveal to others what he is feeling. He has enough insight to recognise his vulnerability to stimuli and impulses. Recognising that this susceptibility can produce trouble for him, he simply holds them inside, not allowing them to be socially visible. This is a fragile strategy; the person is still just as vulnerable and must expend considerable energy keeping himself under control.

As the pathology progresses into the third stage, the inefficiency of mind, the poor comprehension, the impulsivity and vulnerability finally result in a paranoid state. The patient feels so vulnerable that he begins to perceive everyone as his enemy. The fragile control mechanism has not succeeded so that inevitably he perceives everyone as an adversary, someone he must defend against.

By this point, the patient is not actually insane, but he may feel he is going insane, and he may have a fear of insanity, particularly at night.

In the final stage of mental pathology, we do not see the development of overt insanity as we see in many remedies. In Mercurius, the lack of reactive power is so extreme that it cannot even generate an insane state. Instead there develops imbecility. It is as if the brain has become softened and incapable of reacting at all. All stimuli are absorbed, but no longer comprehended.

The sequence of events in the development of illness in *Mercurius* on the physical and mental levels both is one of the classic examples of progression of pathology so well understood by the science of homoeopathy. Although *Mercurius* can affect every organ system, we see most commonly that its "target organs" seem

Mercurius Solubilis

to be first the skin and mucous membranes, next the spinal column, and finally the brain. The slow, insidious progression of illness through these organs calls to mind the possibility that *Mercurius* has a particular affinity for ectodermally—derived structures. As is well known to biology, the embryo is differentiated into three derivative tissues; ectoderm, mesoderm, and endoderm. Each of these tissues result in separate functions in the mature organism. The ectodermal structures include in particular the skin, the mucous membranes near the surface of the body, the eyes, and the nervous system. These are structures for which *Mercurius* has an affinity.

The weakness in defensive reaction is evident throughout all the physical symptomatology of *Mercurius*. As mentioned before, Mercurius patients have one of the most narrow ranges of tolerance to heat and cold of all remedies. Because of weakness of the defence mechanism, there is great instability to the Mercurius system. This is evident in a variety of physical symptoms for which Mercurius is well known.

Mercurius is known for easy perspiration, and then not being relieved by it. Perspiration is a normal function designed to cool the body when it is being overheated, and also to excrete toxic products. In *Mercurius*, however, the slightest stimulus or exertion produces perspiration because of his oversensitivity. It is an over-reaction to a minimal stimulus. Then even the perspiration itself becomes a source of aggravation to the person with such a narrow range of tolerance.

The lack of reactive power is the underlying cause for the characteristic mercurius aggravation from suppression of discharges, such as from otorrhoea or other suppurative disorders. In *Mercurius*, such suppression occurs very easily by orthodox treatment. Unlike the healthy defence which eventually has the power to re-establish the discharge in the same or another form, the Mercurius system merely absorbs the morbific influence, allowing it to create pathology at a deeper level.

There is a tendency to chronic suppurations of all kinds, suppurations which can last for many years. There is simply not enough defensive force to eliminate the infection, so a "stalemate" results, until the allopath interferes and suppresses the infection to a deeper level.

There is much ulceration, particularly of the skin and mucous membranes (aphthae) in *Mercurius*. These are phagadenic ulcerations, ulcers which the body does not have the power to heal and therefore allows them to spread insidiously over ever widening areas.

When a suppuration or ulceration is established in *Mercurius*, there is not enough power to heal them, so a progressive decomposition results. This is most evident in degeneration of the gums. The gums break down, causing a loosening of teeth, a formation of pockets of pus, and a very offensive odour. The offensive odours characteristic of *Mercurius* result from the decomposition which is inevitable in a system lacking the power to react.

Just as we see that perspiration occurs from oversensitivity of the system to any burden placed upon it, we also can see a similar process resulting in the Mercurius excessive salivation. The stomach is disrupted by almost any influence, and then even the slightest disturbance in the stomach results in excessive salivation. The salivation can be seen at any time of day or night, but it is most marked during the night, a typical time of aggravation for *Mercurius*. Having such low reactivity, the patient is steadily weakened by all the influences during the day, until finally the weakness becomes most evident at night; bone pains, the inflammatory symptoms, the nervous system complaints, the fear of insanity, and the salivation are all worse at night.

As an intermediate stage in its progression from the surface of the body to the brain, the Mercurius pathology strikes the spine and peripheral nervous system, producing a tremor, seen particularly in the hands. Such a tremor may frequently be diagnosed as being caused by Parkinson's disease or arteriosclerosis, but its more fundamental cause in a Mercurius case is the defencive weakness and consequent instability of function. The patient finds that he is unable to hold a glass of water in his hands without spilling it, unless he braces his elbow or forearm. This tremor is distinctively symbolic of the Mercurius essence. The lack of reactivity— the weakness in the face of all stimuli which are absorbed easily into the system—results finally in an instability in small functions. Just as the temperature control mechanism swings back and forth between slight extremes of heat and cold, vainly trying inefficiently to compensate, so also the

Mercurius Solubilis

hand wavers back and forth in an inefficient attempt to perform its normal function—hence the tremor.

Once this essence of the Mercurius image is comprehended, one can re-read the Materia Medicas and discover that the morass of data now fits into a single coherent picture.

NATRUM MURIATICUM (nat-m.)

The primary characteristic underlying the *Natrum mur.* pathology is introversion arising out of a feeling of great vulnerability to emotional injury. Natrum mur. patients are emotionally very sensitive; they experience the emotional pain of others, and feel that any form of rejection, ridicule, humiliation or grief would be personally intolerable. Consequently, they create a wall of invulnerability, become enclosed in their own worlds, and prefer to maintain control over their circumstances. They avoid being hurt at all costs.

People susceptible to developing the Natrum mur. type of pathology are emotionally sensitive and vulnerable, but quite clear and strong on mental and physical levels. Mentally, they have a high degree of objectivity and awareness, as well as a great sense of responsibility. For this reason, they are likely to be the sympathetic ear to whom others turn when distressed. The emotional sensitivity and the sense of responsibility readily lead such people into fields of counselling, psychotherapy, the ministry etc. While listening sympathetically to someone else's suffering, such people maintain their objectivity and appear to be very strong. They internally absorb the pain of others, however, and they dwell on it later; particularly, they wonder "How would I react in such a situation? Would I be able to take it".

Throughout life, individuals with Natrum mur. tendencies experience deeply all impressions of life, accumulating awareness and understanding beyond their age. They are strong and enjoy being presented with challenging circumstances, even those involving emotional risk. At first, they enjoy company and thrive on the nourishment of emotional contact with others. They enjoy receiving affection from others—indeed, they inwardly expect and demand it, even though they do not themselves express affection easily. They are so sensitive that they feel hurt by the slightest comment or gesture that might imply ridicule or rejection. Natrum mur. adolescents, for example are reluctant to date, for fear of rejection. Even imagined slights can cause suffering. After being hurt several times, they learn to become cautious. They

Natrum Muriaticum

will think twice before becoming involved in an emotional experience. They turn to introverted activities which are emotionally "safe", i.e. reading books (usually romantic fiction or things having practical value in human relations), listening to music, dwelling on ideas and fantasies.

They can become quite content in their isolation. They tend to be self-contained, desiring to solve problems by themselves without trusting help from other people. Gradually, they come to the point of not needing contact with the outside world. If someone intrudes upon their private, introverted world, they may feel resentful. Their primary concern in life becomes, "not to hurt and not to be hurt".

The issue of emotional pain, in themselves or in others, would be the end of the world for them, they are completely incapable of knowingly inflicting pain on others. For this reason, they become very serious. They cannot make jokes that might inadvertently ridicule someone else. They may appear cold and overly objective to others because they are so intent on not revealing their own emotional vulnerability or creating injury to others. This, combined with the Natrum mur. sense of responsibility, results in guilt being a strong motivating factor in the lives of such people.

Physically, children with Natrum mur. tendencies are likely to be thin and delicate. It is common to see a fine, precise horizontal line dividing the lower eyelid in two. This line is commonly seen in young girls with hysterical personalities; other remedies showing this line include Asafoetida, Lilium tig., and Moschus. In addition, there may be a characteristic crack in the middle of the lower lip.

A Natrum mur. child is very sensitive to disharmony. If the parents fight the child may not react immediately but will suffer inside, perhaps even to the point of acquiring a physical ailment.

These children are usually quite well-behaved; it is not necessary to severely discipline them because a mere glance conveying disapproval will suffice.

The hysterical tendency in Natrum mur. children is seen readily when they are severely reprimended. They then react to an extreme degree, falling on the floor in a tantrum, kicking and screaming. Consolation or reassurance are of no avail, and may acutally make them worse; they will continue with the tantrum until they themselves decide to stop.

At an older age, the hysterical tendency shows itself in another way. Ordinarily, Natrum mur. people do not express emotion readily; they do not cry easily, for example, when suffering a grief. They may be quite serious in their demeanour. However, when nervous or under stress, they tend to laugh over serious matters, then to giggle hysterically; as this giggling becomes uncontrollable, it dissolves into hysterical weeping.

Adolescents of this type are likely to be quiet and withdrawn, but with a sense of responsibility and integrity. At a party, they tend to sit on the sidelines, enjoying themselves by watching others and imagining what they are experiencing. If they are attracted to someone, they will not be flirtatious or friendly. Indeed, they may appear to pay no attention at all, only watching the other out of the corner of the eye. They are liable to fantasize that the other person is likewise attracted and they may romantically blow the entire situation out of proportion. This is the reason why Kent states that a young girl who needs Natrum mur. will easily fall in love with a married man, or someone unattainable. This then causes intense anguish and grief, and the result is an even greater introversion.

They develop intense emotional and sentimental attachments for people, but they don't show their feelings. A daughter may have a deep feeling for her father without anyone else realising it. Then the father dies. The daughter grieves silently, locking herself in her room and crying in her pillow. To the surprise of everyone around her who did not realise the depth of her affection, she becomes very introverted, desiring only to be alone with her books and her music. There is no moaning or crying in front of others—merely occasional sighing perhaps. This internal state continues until she finally breaks down. Then there is uncontrolled, hysterical sobbing with massive shaking of the body, spasms, and twitchings. Such an outburst usually lasts just a short time, and she quickly regains control and composure.

The first stage of pathology in Natrum mur. appears on the physical level. There may be gastritis, arthritis, migraine headaches, canker sores, or herpes on the lower lip. As might be expected, such conditions are likely to occur after a period of introversion following a sever grief or humiliation.

Alternatively, the patient may become hysterically reactive to every influence in the environment—overly sensitive to noise, to light, to cigarette smoke, etc. In such patients, allergies and eczema are common.

Neurological disorders are also very common in Natrum mur. Neuralgias affecting the left eye or the left intercostal nerves, for example, are frequent. Multiple sclerosis often responds to Natrum mur. as well, when the totality of symptoms fits. Heart disease can occur, but it tends to mainfest as arrhythmias and palpitations—which arise from the influence of the nervous system on the heart.

It is during the earliest phases of pathology that some of the most well-known Natrum mur. keynotes are found. The patient has a strong desire for salt, and an aversion to slimy food and to fat, there is an aversion to chicken as well. Characteristically, there is an intolerance to heat, sensitivity to light, and aggravation (of headaches and skin particularly) from the sun. These are true to varying degrees in all of the *Natrums*, but they are more or less equally expressed in *Natrum mur*. The *Natrum mur.* aggravations from the sun and light are not as marked as they are in *Natrum sulph.* and its aggravation from the sun is not as marked as in Natrum carb. The Natrum mur. patient may be sensitive to both heat and to cold, though usually more so to heat. It is less sensitive to heat than Natrum sulph., and also less sensitive to cold than *Natrum carb.*

A characteristic symptom of *Natrum mur.* is the inability to pass urine or stool in the presence of others. This arises from the fear of ridicule, resulting in a chronic tension of sphincter muscles which can be relaxed only in private.

As the emotional vulnerability becomes increasingly pathological the patient becomes depressed. This is a depression which is inconsolable, and may even become suicidal. Suppose, for example, a young man experiences a severe rejection or grief; he retires to his room and puts on the saddest music he can find. The music is not designed to alleviate the depression, but rather to add to it. He wallows in the depression. If one thing has gone wrong, he exaggerates everything out of all proportion. He allows no-one to help; he tries to solve the problem within himself. Eventually, when the depression begins to pass, he regains a more appropriate perspective on life, and music will at that point relieve the remnants of the depression. It is in this sense that music may be either aggravation or amelioration to *Natrum mur.*, depending on the circumstances.

This kind of depression is a kind of hysterical reaction. Ordinarily, the Natrum mur. patient is objective as long as control over the emotions is maintained; but when emotional control breaks down, the patient becomes irrational, and the emotional sphere rules everything.

As the pathology moves beyond the phase of depression, the patient begins to experience periodicity of physical symptoms and alternation of moods.

Physical complaints occur at predictable intervals and times. This is why *Natrum mur.* is often indicated in patients who have suffered from malaria in the past or who have been adversely affected by quinine drugs; it also can be useful in patients in whose family there has been malaria. Migraine attacks often seen in Natrum mur. patients tend to occur at fixed times, usually between 10 a.m. and 3 p.m. Asthmatic attacks, likewise, tend to occur between 5 and 7 p.m.

The moods swing from unreasonable depression to unreasonable exhilaration. As the patient's objectivity becomes interfered with, everything on the emotional level is carried to extremes.

By this stage, some of the characteristic physical symptoms may gradually disappear. As the pathology progresses to deeper levels, there may no longer be desire for salt, aversion to slimy or fatty foods, aggravation from the sun, etc. The disappearance of these traits is directly proportional to the progressive deepening of the pathological state. Often it will be necessary for the homoeopath to inquire into such symptoms not only in the present, but also the past.

As the pathology begins to reach into the emotional level, the first fear that develops in claustrophobia. In early stages, Natrum mur. patients enjoy relative emotional freedom and resent any constrictions imposed by others. Later on, their own vulnerability causes them to close off. When they perceive the same kind of enclosure outside themselves (i.e. closed or narrow places) as

Natrum Muriaticum

they have created within, they become fearful.

Along with the claustrophobia, there occurs a rigidification of the emotional and mental planes. The patient develops fixed ideas; things are seen in terms of good or bad, right or wrong, correct or incorrect, practical or impractical.

Eventually, a hypochondriacal anxiety about health emerges, particularly in regard to heart disease. This hypochondriasis is related to the fastidiousness seen in Natrum mur. The patient is driven by a compulsive need to avoid contamination—always cleaning washing hands, disinfecting everything. In *Natrum mur.* fastidiousness is specifically a fear of microbial contamination, and not so much the feeling of disgust seen in other remedies (*Sulph, Puls, Merc, Phos, Mezereum*). Also, in *Natrum mur.* anxiety about health is much less significant than hypochondriasis, which is more of an anxiety—compulsive attention to details about health.

Finally, even the compulsive control mechanisms break down completely, and the person openly expresses everything which previously had been disallowed. They become shameless, exhibitionistic, speak in obscenities, etc. In the final stage, Natrum mur. patients do not usually lose mental control to the point of developing full-blown insanity, but shameless behaviour may occur.

Naturm mur. is such a deep-acting remedy, and it is so commonly indicated in our western world, that there are many other remedies to which it should be compared.

Ignatia, of course, is the closest of all remedies to *Natrum mur*. In many respects, they are virtually identical. For this reason, they often replace one another in particular cases. Generally, *Ignatia* acts more superficially and is more likely to be indicated in cases where patients' reactions are more superficial. Natrum mur. patients have greater strength, they can tolerate more emotional stress and more intense shocks without breaking down. In Ignatia, the person breaks down with relatively minor stress. In addition, the Ignatia pathology does not as readily affect the physical level. Thus. *Ignatia* is more indicated in emotional reactions appearing after ordinary griefs experienced in life, whereas *Natrum mur.* is more commonly indicated in instances of extraordinary stresses, particularly those causing breakdown on the physical level.

The Ignatia patient frequently feels constricted in the throat or in breathing, especially following an emotional shock. The characteristic Ignatia sighing is an attempt to relieve this sensation of constriction. *Ignatia* cries more easily and is more likely to cry during the homoeopathic interview than *Natrum mur.* Following a grief, the Ignatia patient is less likely to experience sleeplessness than *Natrum mur.*

Frequently, particularly when there are mostly physical symptoms, *Phosphorus* may be difficult to differentiate from Natrum mur. Physically, both look quite similar—thin, sensitive, even perhaps hyperthyroid. The main point of differentiation, of course, is whether the patient has a personality which is closed or open. The sensitive person who tends to be more withheld and evasive, who leans back in the chair while describing symptoms, is more likely to need *Natrum mur.* The Phosphorus patient, on the other hand, is very open and expressive of emotion, tending to lean forward and engage the interviewer in personal contact.

Lilium tig. is a highly hysterical remedy, as is *Natrum mur.* If a Lilium tig. patient experiences rejection or humiliation, however, there is an instantaneous, impulsive reaction; the Natrum mur. patient on the other hand, will suffer inside and wait quite a long time before finally breaking down into a hysterical reaction. *Lilium tig.* is also more likely to be malicious and cruel during such a reaction, whereas the Natrum mur. person would rather inflict suffering on himself than cause pain to anyone else.

Moschus is another hysterical remedy, but the diffenentiation is quite easy. This type of hysteria is designed for others to observe. It is manipulative, an attempt to emotionally blackmail others into a desired response. *Natrum mur.* would rather hide any reaction as much as possible.

Pulsatilla is sometimes confused with *Natrum mur.* Both are intolerant to heat aggravated in the sun, and averse to fat. *Pulsatilla*, however, is emotionally highly expressive, automatically giving affection. When a Pulsatilla patient cries (which occurs easily), it is a "sweet" gentle crying, whereas the Natrum mur. weeping is a spasmodic, loud sobbing which shakes the whole body. Pulsatilla patients that are suffering will actively seek help from others and depend on them; *Natrum mur.* is more self-reliant, preferring to solve problems by themselves.

Natrum Muriaticum

Lycopodium is a remedy which displays an outer shell created in reaction to an inner state, but internally it is, weak and cowardly. *Natrum mur.* is strong, but emotionally vulnerable to being hurt. *Sepia* is closely related to *Natrum mur*. Particularly in children, they may be very difficult to tell apart. Sepia children are very sensitive, and much more excitable than *Natrum mur*. In their excitability, they can become flushed and hyperactive. In adulthood, it is as if the Sepia patient has been broken down by this excessive excitability, becoming fatigued, mentally dulled, and apathetic, *Natrum mur*. feels affection but does not express it easily; Sepia fundamentally has lost it. The Sepia patient is much more likely to be malicious and cruel, almost enjoying hurting others; this would be unthinkable for *Natrum mur*.

NITRIC ACID (*nit-ac.*)

It is difficult to find a single word that encompasses the Nitric acid patient, but if I were to choose one it would be, "pests", the effect the Nitric acid patient has on others due to the constant internal state of DISSATISFACTION; these patients are always dissatisfied and miserable. They are never pleased, even under the most joyful circumstances. In this way they reach a state where they are considered unfit for company by others; they are not at all enjoyable to be with and this is why others call them "pests".

Let us consider the different stages of Nitric acid pathology, which displays an intricate intertwining of the physical, emotional and mental planes. The most prominent aspect of the physical pathology is a SLUGGISHNESS of the circulation. This underlies many of the elements in the Nitric acid picture. It is responsible for the extreme weakness seen in *Nitirc acid*, as well as the marked chilliness. It also causes indolent ulcers which keeps on oozing and spreading. Another characterisitic of *Nitric acid* is the fissures found at the junctions of skin and mucous membranes. These can be attributed to dryness in these areas which causes the skin to crack easily. Physiologically, this dryness can be explained by the sluggish circulation.

It seems that the kidneys and other internal organs of elimination do not function efficently in *Nitric acid*, and therefore a lot of waste products must be eliminated through the skin—generally through discharges. That is why the Nitric acid patient is an OFFENSIVE patient in general. There is very offensive perspiration of the feet. Even the urine smells like that of a horse. Discahrges are offensive, acrid, corrosive, and very irritating to the patient.

There is a characteristic disturbance of the metabolism in *Nitric acid*. The Nitric acid patient is usually thin and nervy, since he does not easily absorb fat, and consequently he has a craving for fat. He also desires strong food which is spicy, and salty fish such as herring. There is cracking in the jaw when chewing.

The Nitric acid patient, as Kent mentions, has an amelioration from riding in a carriage. Of course, this feature is rarely

Nitric Acid

observed today with our smooth cars. I believe it is actually an amelioration from gentle vibrations of the whole body, a steady vibration which ameliorates by gently stimulating the circulation.

Physically, Nitric acid patients look anaemic, with sunken pale skin, especially in the face. The expression is haggard and anxious. Nitric acid patients, because of their general weakness, give the impression that their health is deteriorating rapidly. In the early stages, symptoms are mostly on the physical level, the patient does not bring out any of the great anxiety about health which is produced in later stages. He says,"Never mind if I die", but INTERNALLY he is quite worried that eventually his health is going to break down. This internal feeling, together with the physical weakness, gives him a sense of defeat in regard to his health. He eventually reaches the conclusion that nothing can be done for him. Thus, there is a kind of despair of recovery in Nitric acid, though not as prominent or as clear as we see in Calcarea or Arsenicum.

As always, it is important to recall that once the symptomatology enters on the deeper planes, many of the physical symptoms may disappear. Once the anxiety over health and fear of death become a constant torment, we may no longer get the odour from the feet, or the desires for both fat and salt, even if they have not been already suppressed as being "bad for health". The physical symptoms disappear in proportion to the increase in fears and anxieties.

The Nitric acid individual has an unrestful sleep, he wakes up in the morning feeling very cross, very irritable, and very tired. Each of the main remedies for unrefreshing sleep has its own unique qualities. Nitric acid is so irritable at this time of day that nobody can even greet him. I remember a Nitric acid case who was working in a shop. The customers, of course, would come in and say "Good morning." He would merely mumble a grudging "Morn...". It is too difficult for him to speak in the morning. Everything looks very dark and desperate for *Nitric acid* in the morning. The pains, on the other hand, are all aggravated at night; the splinter-like pains, arthritic pains, and the pains in the long bones.

Turning now to the emotional pathology, we see in the *Nitric acid* an "anxiety neurosis". Kent talks about the great sensitivity of this patient. It is an internal sensitivity. Everything bothers him, nothing satisfies him. Noise can bother such a patient, but it is not only noise, even little disturbances which he has in the physical body become great annoyances. In this way, the internal sensitivity is seen to be more of a chronic state of dissatisfication and unhappiness. Cap this with irritability, and we have the picture of Nitric acid.

They are always complaining. Some may complain openly to other people, whereas many turn their complaints inward. These latter people develop a kind of UNFORGIVENESS. It is very characteristic of Nitric acid that he cannot forget a wrong done to him. If the wrong-doer says, "I am sorry. I was wrong. It was in a moment of irritablity that I told you those things." The Nitric acid patient will say, "Yes, yes, it is alright, I do not care." But inside he will never forgive him. This is a symptoms that we can find even in the first stages, in which the pathology is in the physical body.

We see then an individual who has been disappointed by the world and who has no courage to continue fighting. He lives as if he is just drifting with the flow, feeling that nothing matters. This is a state of apathy and indifference . It is in this way that the original weakness spreads throughout the three levels, finally reaching a state of great isolation. His feelings become bland. He develops a philosophy to excuse this state. He becomes a nihilist, not believing in anything. He seems to have no force to start something new, no initiative for anything. He has lost hope and urge to do things.

To summarise the psychology of the Nitric acid person; such a person is irritable. He is sensitive both inside and outside: inside because of his own thoughts, and outside because of every little injury he thinks people do to him, noises, or other disturbances. He is unahappy, unsatisfied, unforgiving. He is so engrossed in his own misery and dissatisfiaction that he cannot see anything outside himself.

Within the first stages of pathology, there are mainly physical complaints and weakness, but on occasion the patient may experience strongly a fear of death. As the pathology progresses, we see that development of a tremendous anxiety about health. Even more commonly, however, is the anxiety about health that occurs

Nitric Acid

in an entirely different **Nit. acid patient.** Usually the pathological anxiety about health comes about in people who have been living quite comfortably—the "dolce vita" jet-setters—and then suddenly the doctor suggests that some minor complaints needs checking to rule out something serious. From this moment on they become panicky, and this anxiety about their health may remain for a very long time unless they get Nitric acid.

This is completely insane anxiety. For example, a Nitric acid woman finds a pimple on her scalp and she quickly decides that there is about a 90% chance that it is cancer of the brain. You explain to her that cancer of the brain developes inside the skull, not outside, but she still is not satisfied. She goes to another doctor, and then to a third, and a fourth. She is one of those patients who keeps on telephoning the doctor all the time, arguing, "Yes, I see your point, the pimple is going away anyway, but now I have a **little pain in the left side of my chest.**This must be cancer...." The main anxiety in Nitric acid is for cancer. They do not fear so much heart disease orstroke, their fear is for terminal ailment such as cancer which they believe inevitably leads to death.

Another feature of Nitric acid patients is that they do not esily make contact with others. They talk as there IS ALWAYS A BARRIER between them and others. Even when there is anxiety and the doctor confirms that nothing is wrong, they remain absolutely certain of their own idea. It is as if this barrier prevents any real communication. Nitric acid patients stay within their own world of suspicion. Because of this, these people make very poor conversationalists;they seem incapable of seeing the point of the other person.

EXCITABILITY IN SEX is another feature of Nitric acid. The Nitric acid man is likely to be the type who often visits **Prostitutes**, having sex purely out of physical excitability, and not caring about emotional or mental contact. It is not actually that he does not care, but he has decided that he cannot find a woman perfect enough to suit him. So he chooses instead to have sexual inter**course only on a physical level.**

Eventually, the pathology reaches into the mental sphere. Nitric acid patients may dwell on thoughts of suicide because they can find no way to make it in the world. They feel too weak to cope with circumstances, and as a result there is finally the thought of suicide. However, due to the great fear of death, they are normally too afraid to kill themselves. I remember a case in which the patient came to the interview with a pistol in his pocket. He readily confessed to me that he had decided to commit suicide. He was carrying the pistol around just waiting for the right moment to use it. He had been carrying it for months. Finally, he got Nitric acid, and sold his pistol. I remember that he had severe acne—a kind of malignant acne such as we usually see with Cal. sulph., or Calc. silicata. He had the typical morning aggravation of *Nitric acid*. He was so averse to talking to anyone during the first hour or so in the morning that he felt capable of literally killing someone for saying a simple, "Good morning."

Sometime you will have to get this information from the relatives. You cannot get it straight from the patient because he does not realise that his disease has become a philosophy for him. He thinks to himself, "Why should I greet anyone in the morning?" He has decided what life is, and he sees no other point of view. It is not a limitation of freedom that is perceived by the patient. Despite all this, the worst state this patient is likely to reach is the fear of death. It is not a remedy that would be indicated in real insanity.

NUX VOMICA (nax-v.)

Nux vomica is one of the more commonly prescribed remedies in the homoeophathic Materia Medica, being one of the remedies absolutely essential for every homoeopath to know in depth. To begin with, we will describe the type of person most commonly affected by *Nux*, and then describe in more depth the peculiar Nux vomica pathology. Generally, the, Nux person possesses a husky, solid, compact, muscular body type, a basically strong constitution. They are ambitious, intelligent, quick, capable and competent. Frequently, their upbringing emphasises a strong sense of duty, and strongly values the work ethic. The Nux person is self-reliant rather than dependent. Their intelligence is pragmatic and efficient rather than philosophical or intellectual. The Nux person in the non-pathological state, makes an excellent, hard-working, efficient employee—and their talents lead them toward such occupations as supervisors, managers, businessmen, accountants, salesmen.

As always in homoeopathy, however, we must be careful not to prescribe *Nux vomica* on the basis of such positive and constructive personality traits. Unlike the techniques of astrology, palmistry, handwriting analysis, physiognomy and others, which describe the qualities of the person—whether for good or bad—homoeopathy bases its prescriptions on the pathological state of the person. We would not wish to give a remedy which might make a person less pragmatic and efficient! So, let us consider the states in the develoment of the pathological state requiring *Nux vomica* for cure.

In the first stage, the Nux person demonstrates an exaggeration, an excess of the normally beneficial qualities of ambition and conscientiousness. Instead of using their talents merely at work in an appropriate, relaxed and balanced manner, the Nux person begins to become ruled by them. The ambition begins to occupy him during all the hours of the day and night, becoming a driving ambition, an over-emphasis on achievement and competition. *Nux* is the most competitive remedy in the Materia Medica, competitive to the point of damaging his own health and even at the expense of his colleagues. the Nux person can become a workaholic dominated by work. Because he is capable and efficient, it is likely that he will be rapidly promoted to greater and greater responsibilities. The Nux person will welcome such promotions. Two other remedies with similar physical symptomatologies, Arsenicum and Phosphorus, will take different attitudes. Arsenicum will tend to decline a promotion with too much responsibility, partially because the self-centred Arsenicum person is more interested in personal comfort than achievement. The Phosphorus patient may be intelligent and quick also, but will shrink from the intense competitiveness which might be necessary to get ahead.

In Nux vomica, the normally conscientious state can be exaggerated out of proportion, leading to a compulsive efficiency. Nux is one of only a few remedies listed under the rubric Fastidious, but specifically the Nux fastidiousness is tied to the emphasis on efficiency. In this sense, the Nux fastidiousness is more appropriate to reality and not so severely pathological as would be assumed by its designation in italics in the Repertory. The Arsenicum fastidiuousness, on the other hand, is a typcal example of the severe neurotic, syphilitic fastidiousness so classically described by psychiatrists. It is a compulsively neurotic concern with cleanliness and order, both arising out of a deep-seated, anguished feeling of insecurity; the Arsenicum patient is constantly straightening and cleaning, far in excess of what is required for simple efficiency. *Natrum mur.* is another well-known fastidious remedy; in this case, it is more a concern with punctuality and scheduling of time.

Eventually, the Nux vomica person may end up in a job which is over his head. Typically, he responds by working harder and longer, expecting more from himself and others. The Nux person characteristically carries the implicit assumption that any challenge, any problem, can be overcome by sheer effort and ability. One of the most difficult things for a Nux patient to do is to accept a limitation, or to resign himself to the inevitable. To keep up with the pressure, he comes to use various artificial means to keep himself stimulated, coffee, cigarettes, drugs (whether by prescription or social drugs such as marijuana), alcohol, and even sex. Despite such abuse of stimulants, it is also true that Nux patients are also unusually sensitive to many of these substances

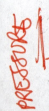

and consequently suffer consequences of their indulgences.

The Nux vomica person is known to be a hyper-sexual individual. They have a very strong sexual desire, and may indulge their sexual impulses even beyond the bounds of conventional morality. Despite being bound by the work ethic, the Nux person is not the typical upright, moralistic personality. In their use of stimulants and drugs, and most particularly in their sexual sphere, their behaviour is conducted out of impulse and therefore is best described as "amoral". As in the rest of the Nux picture, the over indulgence of sex finally results in a state of exhaustion; in later stages, the Nux patient suffers from impotence, typically a loss of erection upon intromission.

The over-indulgence of stimulants may meet his needs for a while, but eventually, the over-stimulation and toxicity take their toll. The stomach becomes disordered. The entire nervous system becomes overwhelmed and oversensitive. Even slight stresses such as light, small noises, someone's voice or singing becomes intolerable. The effects of the "over-amped" nervous system are described brilliantly by Kent; "For example, a businessman has been at his desk until he is tired out, he received many letters, he has a great many irons in the fire; he is troubled with a thousand little things; his mind is constantly hurried from one thing to another until he is tortured. It is not so much the heavy affairs but the little things. He is compelled to stimulate his memory to attend to all the details; he goes home and thinks about it; he lies awake at night; his mind is confused with the whirl of business and the affairs of the day crowd upon him; finally, brain-fag comes on. When the details come to him he gets angry and wants to get away, tears things up, scolds, goes home and takes it out on his family and children. Sleeps by fits and starts; wakens at 3 a.m. and his business affairs crowd on him so that he cannot sleep again until late in the morning when he falls into a fatiguing sleep and wakens up tired and exhausted. He wants to sleep late in the morning."

The Nervous system seems to become bound up, works against itself. Again, this is described best by Kent; "Another state running through Nux is that actions are turned in opposite directions. When the stomach is sick, it will empty its contents with no great effort ordinarily, but in *Nux* there is retching and straining as if the action were going the wrong way, as if it would force the abdomen open; a reversed action; retches, gags and strains, and after a prolonged effort he finally empties the stomach. The same condition is found in the bladder. He must strain to urinate. There is tenesmus, urging. The bladder is full and the urine dribbles away, yet when he strains it ceases to dribble. In regard to the bowels, though the patient strains much, he passes but a scanty stool. In the diarrhoea at times when he sits on the commode in a perfectly passive way, there will be a little squirt of stool, and then comes on tenesmus so that he cannot stop straining, and when he does strain, there comes on the sensation of forcing back; the stool seems to go back; a kind of anti-peristalsis. In constipation the more he strains the harder it is to pass a stool."

These are the patients complaining of gastritis or ulcer or "spastic colon". They finally go to the doctor, who pronounces their condition psychosomatic and prescribes antiacids, antispasmodics, tranquillisers, or even psychotherapy. These merely mask the symptom, usually ineffectively, and consequently worsen the sensitivity of the nervous system in general.

The Nux patient, then, is very irritable, but this is a kind of irritability which the homoeopath may find difficult to elicit without care. The Nux patient will tend to hold the irritability inside (at least in this early stage). You ask, "Are you irritable?" The patient says, "No not at all. I never even raise my voice." So you ask, "How about inside? Do you feel irritable inside yourself?" Patient; "Oh yes! Very much!!" It is such people, who are most prone to gastritis and peptic ulcer. If the person were to learn to be more expressive, he would be spared the ulcer—but then, the abuse of coffee, cigarettes, and alcohol might result in the same condition, anyway.

Finally, the pressures become too much and the Nux patient becomes impatient and irritable. He becomes impatient with himself, and particularly with others, scolding and reproaching others over minor incidents. He reacts impulsively over small disturbances. Someone quietly whistles a tune, and he yells "Can't you keep quiet!" He can't find a pencil, so he slams the desk drawer shut. He has momentary difficulty buttoning his shirt, so he rips the button off. Someone contradicts him, and he stalks out of the

Nux Vomica

room while loudly slamming the door. He is intolerant to contradiction, but not so much from arrogance or haughtiness (like Lycopodium or Platinum), but rather because he is certain he is right and is impatient with others who have not thought the problem through as quickly or as thoroughly as he; and, indeed, he is most often right. His impulsivity can lead to many personnel difficulties; Nux vomica patients are blunt and undiplomatic, and therefore would not make very good politicians by nature.

In the next stage of development, Nux becomes actually malicious, cruel, violent. Cruelty may begin by talking behind the backs of others, particularly arising out of impulse, kicking animals (Like medorrhinum). As this progresses, Nux may become outright violent; most likely, many husbands who beat their wives, or parents who commit child abuse would benefit from Nux, (if the rest of the image fits, of course). The violence is not necessarily focussed always on others; Nux also can have a suicidal disposition, particularly by shooting himself with a gun or jumping from a height.

The final stage of Nux is a state of insanity, a paranoid state. The Nux patient is constantly tormented by the impulse to kill others, but may not manifest actual violence. A woman may be haunted by a desire to throw her baby into the fire, or to kill her husband. In the Repertory *Nux* is listed under a variety of delusions having to do with murder, being murderded, being injured or insulted, and of failure. To the external observer, however, the internal torment of the Nux patient may not be at all evident. This is the stage when Nux has an aversion to company and refuses to answer questions. It is a state of mental disorder which may appear very much like that described in the last stage of Arsenicum; although a careful history of the stages of the development of the pathology will make the distinction very clear. Nux is self-reliant, independent, compulsively hard-working, overly efficient, and irritable and impulsive; while *Arsenicum* is insecure, dependent concerned about personal health and comfort, compulsive about cleanliness and order, and very anxious.

Considering the physical level of the Nux image, a general impression is that Nux vomica primarily affects functional difficulties. It does not have the deep degenerations that are characteristic, for example, in Arsenicum, which has deep spreading ulcerations and gangrenous putrefactions.

Nux vomica affects very strongly the nervous system. There are initially many twitchings and jerkings, similar to those in Hyoscyamus and Agaricus. There are severe neuralgic pains, particularly of the head. Nux is often needed in apopleptic states, expecially in cases in which the paralysis is accompanied by sticking pains in the affected limbs. In more extreme disorders, there are convulsions, opisthotonos, epilepsies. Considering the abuse of stimulants like alcohol, it is not suprising that Nux vomica is a remedy which might be indicated in delirium tremens.

All beginning students of homoeopathy are taught the generalities of Nux vomica; chilly, worse from drafts, worse in the morning. Nux is one of the chilliest of remedies; however, it tends specifically to be more aggravated in cold, dry environments and ameliorated in wet weather (along with Asarum, Causticum and Hepar sulph). Nux is very sensitive to drafts, which can easily cause a coryza if the patient has perspired (which occurs easily in Nux from slight exertion). A peculiar characteristic of Nux coryzas is that the nose is stuffed up while outdoors and flows fluently indoors; also, the nose runs freely during daytime and stuffs up at night.

The gastrointestinal tract is particularly sensitive in *Nux*. As mentioned, gastritis and peptic ulcer are commonly seen, causing spasms, eructations, gagging and retching, which are unsatisfying to the patient. There is great sensitivity to almost all kinds of food; in the broken down Nux state, especially there will be little appetite, and the patient will be found to be a very picky eater. There is an aversion to meat, yet there may be a desire for fat—as well as for stimulants, pungent things, and spices, which are craved for the stimulating effects but which may disorder the stomach. The Nux patient will report that he bocomes sick whenever his stomach is disordered; he gets a cold, a headache or asthma. Pains in the abdomen are commonly accompanied by the desire for stool which so frustrates Nux.

As is commonly seen in alcoholics, the Nux system may show congestion of the portal system—oesophageal varices, and particularly haemorrhoids. There is also a tendency to jaundice, corresponding in many instances to cirrhosis of the liver. Nux will sometimes relieve the spasm of gallstone colic, enabling the stone to pass into the intestinal tract; it may also relieve renal stone colic in the same manner.

In conclusion, it is important to be reminded that the symptoms described in this paper are not designed to be exhaustive, but merely to present an image, to point to the "essence". In any given patient, any combination of such symptoms may be there, perhaps excluding some classic symptoms of Nux, and yet the patient will still require this remedy. In most cases the obsession with tasks or work, the irritability from the over-extended nervous system, and the chilliness will be there. But, for example, a particular patient may avoid alcohol and dislike cigarettes and yet still need *Nux vomica*. In homoeopathic prescribing, we are not matching symptoms per se; rather, we are matching the essence of the patient with the essence of the remedy.

PHOSPHORICUM ACIDUM (*ph-ac.*)

Phosphoric acid is characterised by great weakness or enfeeblement which begins on the emotional plane and progresses subsequently to the physical and mental planes. Prolonged grief or sudden, severe grief are the usual exciting causes. My clinical experience does not bear out Kent's description of mental enfeeblement being the primary pathological state in Phosphoric acid. In patients I have seen, the enfeeblement seems to affect primarily the emotional level, with subsequent progression to either the physical of mental level depending on the hereditary strength or weakness of the constitution.

Innner or outer stimuli can create weakness in every individual at some point—whether on the physical, emotional, or mental levels. The precise level of vulnerability is a matter of individuality. The specific Phosphoric acid weakness begins on the emotional level. By contrast, two other acids primarily affect the other levels; Picric acid leads all remedies by susceptibility to mental enfeeblement, while Muriatic acid is primarily characterised by muscular enfeeblement.

In Phosphoric acid, there is usually a history of grief. This may be grief of a minor nature over a prolonged period of time, or it may be a sudden major grief. In Phosphoric acid, it is not necessary for the grief to be of great intensity; Ignatia, by contrast, requires a greater shock than Phosphoric acid to experience pathology. Characteristically, the phosphoric acid patient suffers the grief in silence—it should be listed in italics in the Repertory under Silent Grief, alongside Ignatia, Natrum mur., and Pulsatilla. The patient's initial response is a kind of softening, or a dropping down in tone on the emotional plane. This then leads to emotional indifference. The patient becomes isolated, wants to be left alone, much like Sepia. The isolationism is even typified by the Phosphoric acid tendency to sleep facing the wall in bed.

As the patient is affected deeper by the grief, the emotional level becomes completely "frozen down"; there is no emotional movement whatsoever. Such a profound stillness occurs on the emotional plane that the patient is incapable of response; it is as if stimuli are not received by the organism at all. The Phosphoric acid patient himself knows he is devoid of emotional responsiveness, even if this is not yet apparent to others around him. Just as there is stillness and coldness physically, there is no movement at all emotionally. This state is similar to Aurum and Sepia. In Aurum, there is a deep inner stillness, a deadening, but this is due to profound depression. The Aurum patient has given up, but still has emotions; it is not a true apathy. In Sepia, there is apathy, but it occurs primarily because of a neutralisation of opposing forces rather than from debility following grief; Sepia patients may feel no emotion in their daily existences, but they can be quickly roused if approached in specific ways. Phosphoric acid patients, on the other hand, are unrousable, indifferent to any kind of stimulation.

A dramatic personality changes may occur in patients who have undergone a very powerful shock—such as the sudden and unexpected loss of a loved one. In this circumstance, the physical level may be bypassed; instead, the defence mechanism reacts with emotional paralysis or stillness. Someone who was active and full of life becomes withdrawn into himself. This is not due to actual depression, but more to inefficiency of emotions and mind. Such a patient neither wishes to die nor to live. His house is in disorder and dirt piles up on the floor, but he does not want to do anything about it. There may be thoughts of suicide, but he does not have the power to actually carry it out.

After the initial stimulus on the emotional level, degeneration may progress to either the physical level in patients with relatively strong constitutions—or to the mental plane in those with very weak constitutions experiencing a sudden loss. We will begin with consideration of cases focussed primarily on the physical level by the time the homoeopath is consulted. A common story is,"I had been very well—quite healthy and active—until a year ago, but there has been a steady degeneration since." The patient is easily tired, whereas his stamina used to be quite good. Upon further enquiry, it is found that the patient had silently suffered a prolonged grief. To most people, the degree of the grief might seem to be insufficient to explain the severity of subsequent breakdown. A woman may complain that her husband pays too much attention to his mother. Or perhaps she has long suspected her husband of adultry, but she tells no-one of her suspicions.

During the stage of physical breakdown, there may be a wide variety of symptoms. The hair falls out suddenly and rapidly. There may be a marked decline in vision. There might be headaches, especially in the temples, with a boiling sensation in the head. There may be chills followed by flushes with perspiration (this symptom is also common in Gelsemium, which is also physically very tired). Often there is a history of unexplained low-grade fever. similar to Ignatia there is a frequent desire to breathe deeply. There may be flatus. Often there is milkiness in the urine, like small curds, particularly at the end of urination. There may also be indifference to sex, impotency, and premature ejaculation.

Dryness is a common symptom in *Phosphoric acid*. There is dryness of the nose and the eyes. The mouth is dry, with a bitter taste. There is usually a desire for fruits, juicy things, and refreshing things. It is as if the patient were dehydrated.

Considering the extreme physical exhaustion, the physical inertia, the falling of hair, the change in visual acuity, the dehydration, and the sexual weakness, one can conjecture that a basic aspect of the Phosphoric acid pathology arises from hypofunction of the endocrine system—particularly the adrenal and sex glands. In a related fashion, the picture is comparable to the known clinical state of metabolic alkalosis.

During the stage of physical breakdown, few emotional or mental symptoms are evident. There may only be silent grief, and perhaps some fear of heights or vertgo from high places. The patient prefers to be left alone, and there may be some degree of apathy.

During the physical stage, it can be very difficult for the homoeopath to recognise *Phosphoric acid* as the correct remedy. There are a number of remedies which could cover the exhaustion and other physical symptoms—including *Helonius, Muriatic acid,* and others. As basic guidelines, however, one should keep in mind the following physical symptoms, which belong most characteristically to *Phosphoric acid*: weakness in the body, dehydration, desire for fruits and juicy things, decreased sexual energy, and loss of hair.

The next stage of pathological development, whether in patients with slow progression after prolonged grief, or in those in which a powerful shock penetrates immediately into the emotional level, is a weakening and degeneration of the mental faculties. Characteristically, the first mental symptoms to occur are tremendous forgetfulness and weakness of memory, particularly for words. Upon questioning, the patient displays a vacant look, finally answering after one or two minutes. The question registers in the mind of the Phosphoric acid patient, but he or she is unable to find the right word for the answer. This is different from the process seen in *Mercurius*, which is also slow in answering; the *Mercurius* slowness occurs both because the mind does not easily comprehend the question and because it takes a long time to find the right answer. *Phosphorus* is another remedy which answers slowly, but this is because of an irritability, an unwillingness to answer.

After a prolonged period of emotional standstill, there is a further enfeeblement of the entire sphere of mental functioning. Mental activity of any kind becomes profoundly difficult, although usually the Phsophoric acid patient is able to continue working. This is in contrast to the Picric acid patient in whom the first stages of weakness begin on the mental plane, resulting in complete inability to do even simple mental work.

Finally, there is a profound apathy affecting all areas of life. In Phosphoric acid this is not a true insanity but merely a deep lack of interest. Insane patients in whom the apathy becomes complete and total, who merely sit and stare at an object, are more likely to require *Pulsatilla*.

In the end, there is profound stillness of emotions, memory, and the ability to think. At this point, there may be complete disappearance of the characteristic physical symptoms. These patients may be able to perform physical work quite readily, and exertion may even be quite beneficial—in contrast to the first stage of physical symptomatology. The hair no longer falls out; instead, it becomes lustreless and greasy.

There is a lack of mental clarity, a haziness of mind, coupled with deep emotional apathy. The patient says he cannot complete a whole idea; even the attempt makes him tired. He forgets the names of people, places and events of the past. He is unable to digest what he has read.

Phosphoric acid needs to be clearly differentiated from other acids. "Paralysis" is a key theme for *Phosphoric acid, Picric acid,* and *Muriatic acid,* but with emphasis on different levels. In Phosphoric acid the emotional is the initial primary foucs. In Picric acid the weakness begins on the mental level and works down through the emotional to the physical plane. For Picric acid, the exciting cause is exertion of the mind. Picric acid patients can stand very little mental exertion; if they continue to work despite the mental weakness, they are liable to get a headache; this is particularly true of Picric acid children (compare Calc. phos. in this situation). Next follows indifference—not, however, as profound as in Phosphoric acid. Finally, there occurs paralytic weakness in the extremities and in the entire body; this is a result of degeneration of the spinal cord. Another differential point is that *Picric acid* is aggravated by heat, whereas *Phophoric acid* is chilly.

Muriatic acid weakness begins in the physical body. There is a profound weakness of muscles—so much so that the patient slides down in the chair or bed because of sheer lack of muscular power. There is also a weakness or paralysis of the tongue and sphincter muscles. From the physical level, the weakness progresses into the emotional and eventually the mental plane.

PHOSPHORUS (*phos.*)

Diffusion is the theme which runs through the Phosphorus pathology. Diffusion is the process of spreading outward into the environment, like smoke spreading outward into the air, or the colour from a tea bag diffusing uniformly into water. The same happens to the energy, the awareness, the emotions, and even the blood of the Phosphorus patient. It is as if there are no barriers for this—physical, emotional, or mental. Because of this, the Phosphorus patient is vulnerable to all types of influences. On the physical level, we see that almost any injury or stress results in haemorrhage; this occurs because the sheaths of the blood vessels are weak and easily allow the blood to diffuse into surrounding tisssues. On the emotional plane, the Phosphorus patient's emotions freely go out toward others, with little ability of the patient to contain them and protect the self from emotional vulnerability. Mentally, the patient easily forgets himself, even to the degree that awareness can become too diffuse and unfocussed; the patient becomes easily "spaced out."

Let us first describe a person in the healthy state who nevertheless possesses the Phosphorus predilection, which can emerge into a desease state if the defence mechanism becomes overwhelmed by too much stress; in doing so, however, keep in mind that we only prescribe on the pathological symptoms, not on the healthy ones. The Phosphorus pateint physically is usually lean, tall, and delicate in features, hair, skin and hands. As a child, this person is warm, outgoing, affectionate, artistic or musical and very sensitive. The child is very open and impressionable; one can "see through" such a child, whose being is effortlessly manifested, without much reserve. During adolescence, there is a tremendous growth spurt which leads to the typically lean, lanky appearance.

Throughout life, the Phosphorus type person is a warm, friendly extrovert who enjoys friendship and company very much, but also may enjoy solitude to pursue artistic endeavours. Such a person is enjoyable to have around, because he or she is truly sympathetic, freely putting the interest of friends above personal concerns. The Phosphorus person is highly intelligent and refined. There are no secrets for such person; whatever is on his mind he shares freely. Warmth and affection diffuse freely towards friends and even strangers. Much of his or her life revolves around interpersonal relationships. Such a person makes a good politician, the type that pushes for humanitarian causes, or a Phosphorus type may become a sales agent beause he has the ability to sell anything he believes in. The Phosphorus person is very impressionable and will believe anything which is told to him in an area outside of his own competence, then once he has adopted a belief he will be enthusiastic and convincing to others.

Such a person makes an enjoyable patient for the homoeopath because he is impressionable and trusting; the Phosphorus patient believes in what the prescriber tells him and follows directions willingly and with effusive gratitude. Right from the first interview, the patient views the prescriber as a friend, shaking his hand warmly, sitting forward on the seat, and perhaps reaching out to touch the prescriber's hand or wrist when emphasising a point. This patient gives symptoms freely, without holding back. There is a predisposition toward anxieties of various types, but these are relieved easily by just a few reassuring words.

The diffusion of awareness is evident by the fact that the Phosphorus patient is easily startled. All of us can relate to the state of mind of daydreaming; awareness drifts to a far-off place or circumstances. During a daydream, if there is a sudden noise, like a blaring horn, a slamming door, or a burst of thunder, the daydreamer is startled because awareness is pulled suddenly and joltingly back into the immense relaity . This is the state to which the Phosphorus patient is highly susceptible. It is a diffusion of awareness which the patient may not be able to control readily. During a thunderstorm, the normal person will hear a clap of thunder and then easily prepare himself for more; the Phosphorus patient, however, tends to become diffuse automatically, and so will be startled with each noise.

In the first stge of Phosphorus pathology, the physical symptoms usually predominate. In the childish stage of development (whether 5 years or 35 years of age), there may be a tendency to easy haemorrhages. Nosebleeds occur with little provocation. Menses may be profuse and prolonged. The bleeding tends to be bright red in colour. The bleeding tendency is symbolic of the general essence of Phosphorus. What warmth and brightness the Phosphorus patient possesses diffuses freely outward, with little sense of barriers.

It is at this stage that we see the Phosphorus patient who is easily refreshed by sleep. This is understandable when we reflect that sleep is a time when the ordinary effort to maintain immediate physical awareness is relaxed and rested. People who are more controlled and mentalised take a long time to achieve this rest; they must fall into a deep sleep. The Phosphorus patient, on the other hand, is quickly refreshed because his awareness can diffuse in this manner very readily.

During this stage, we also see the characteristic Phosphorus thirst, particularly for cold drinks. If there happens to be burning in the stomach (Phosphorus experiences burning pains internally— a manifestation of warmth), the pains will be relieved cold things; but this lasts only until the drink or food warms in the stomach, and then the stomach may be again aggravated. There is a typical craving for chocolate and sweets. Considering the thirst and the craving for sweets, it is easy to see the Phosphorus predilection for diabetes.

As the physical pathology progresses further, the process of haemorrhage may be evident on deeper levels. There may be painless haemorrhage from the gastrointestinal tract, resulting in an unexpected haematemesis or melaena. There may be bronchitis in an early and mild phase, yet with haemoptysis of bright red blood. There may be haematuria unaccompanied by any other sympotoms. Laboratory tests and x-rays may be done, and nothing found. In these circumstances think of *Phosphorus* as a possiable remedy.

While the physical symptoms predominate, there are few symptoms in the emotional or mental spheres. As the pathology progresses, however, into the second stage, we see a subsidence of the physical symptoms and an increase in anxieties and fears. Of course, there is a true anxiety for the welfare of another, whether friend or stranger. It can be carried to a pathological degree of anxiety, dissipating even the energy of the patient himself. This is the true state of sympathy, whereas other remedies in the same rubric are anxious about others out of a primary motive of self-concern.

There is a strong anxiety about health in *Phosphorus*. The patient becomes so suggestible that even if he hears of someone else with a particular illness, he will be concerned about the possiblity that he also might have that illness. This vulnerability to suggestion, however, is easily assuaged by counter-suggestion; a few reassuring words by the homoeopath, and the patient sighs with relief and is profusely thankful, only to come back when he hears another alarming possibility.

It is during this stage that there is the emergence of many fears. There is fear of the dark, fear of being alone, and fear at twilight. There may be a fear of thunderstorms. At first these anxieties and fears are fairly mild, and still corroborated by thirst and refreshed sleep.

As the third stage emerges, the patient becomes overwhelmed by the anxieties and fears. Whereas before they were mild and manageable by simple reassurance, they gradually occupy more and more of the energy and attention of the patient. The patient finds it increasingly difficult to relax, and anxiety may lead to hyperventilation and resultant imbalances in the pH of the blood. The undercurrent of anxiety and tension prevents relaxation even during sleep; the patient awakes unrefreshed and also with great anxiety (like Lachesis, Graphites and Arsenicum).

Eventually, the continuous anxiety becomes a "free-floating anxiety" with no identifiable cause. There is a fear that something bad will happen which pervades the person's life, like background music. Every possibility is anticipated with fear. There is a fear of impending disease, particularly a fear of cancer (rather than heart disease), but eventually the fear of any impending disease.

Finally, the Phosphorus patient falls into a fear of death, a panic state over the idea that death is imminent. The patient feels like he is dying, especially when he is alone. There is the sensation of fuzziness internally, like bubbles rising and diffusing outward, or that the soul is leaving the body. There is great panic, hyperventilation, excitability and palpitations. This is the point when the patient develops a need for company, becuase of the fear that death is imminent.

Phosphorus

The need for company can be so strong as to drive him to leave his house to find friends to talk to. This is not a need to talk to people about health in particular, as in Arsenicum; rather, Phosphorus just feels the need to talk to anybody about anything, in order to relieve the panic.

As the states of fear increase, many of the other corroborating symptoms on the physical level disappear. There may be no thirst, no craving for salt, and no craving for fish.

Finally, in the fourth stage, the mind breaks down completely. The fears diminish, but the mind degenerates. There is a difficulty in concentration, an inability to think coherently, or an inability to understand what is being said by others. The body and the mind become weak. The patient becomes indifferent to comapany and indifferent to surroundings. The result is a state of senility or imbecility. Another common end result in Phosphorus is a stroke in which many mental faculties are lost.

The final stage can be a very difficult one in which to prescribe because there is a paucity of symptoms to distinguish Phosphorus from other remedies. For this reason, a careful history of the past sequence of events and proper knowledge of the stages of pathology of remedies is crucial to being able to benefit the patient.

Once the essence of Phosphorus is seen, one needs only to confirm the remedy with corroborating symptoms. From experience, some of the most useful are; thirst, desire for salt, desire for fish, desire for chocolate, desire for sweets, worse left side, unable to sleep on the left side, formication of the tips of the fingers, painless loss of voice. In addition, different Phosphorus patients may be either warm blooded or chilly—though not in the same patient.

PLATINUM METALLICUM (*plat.*)

Platina is a remedy which exemplifies the process of perversion of and conflict between normal functions which can occur in a particular type of individual. The Platina patient, on the one hand, is driven by a powerful, excessive sexual desire; on the other hand, she is strongly idealistic and romantic in her amorous relationships. The tension, and eventual conflict, between these two aspects of her nature, the repeated disappointments inevitable for a person of such intensity and sensitivity, leads to the pathology which is the essence of this remedy.

As a general rule, Platina most readily affects a particular personality type. Physically, this person tends to be lean, of dark hair, eyes, and complexion. The face is usually round, with full sensual lips. It most readily affects women of a sensitive nature, at once sensual and idealistic. In children, the Platina type may display the traits of pride and integrity.

The Platina pathology shows itself on two levels, primarily the sexual and the mental. From a young age, the Platina woman feels a strong sexual desire, which can be distractingly intense. Throughout life, and beginning at a young age, there may be great hyperaesthesia of the genitals, leading to masturbation. (Origanum is another remedy which displays masturbation in young girls, but it tends to occur more in childhood between the ages of 3 and 7 years, rather than at puberty). The Platina woman is likely to become involved sexually at a young age, and emotionally she will throw herself wholeheartedly into a sexual relationship, with great romanticism and idealism. To compare it with other remedies, we find that Natrum mur, Sepia, Causticum and Calc.carb. develop sexual relationships generally later in life. On the other hand, sexuality occurs at a quite young age in *Nux vomica*, *Lachesis*, *Coffea cruda*, *Platina* and *Staphysagria*. (The Staphysagria patient is too sesitive emotionally to face a sexual relationship, however, and therefore develops a highly active fantasy life, with early masturbation).

The Platina patient wants the relationship to be as fulfilling emotionally as she desires it to be sexually; unfortunately, her desires are so extremely intense that it is virtually impossible for any man to satisfy them. She then becomes disappointed, and begins a process of going from one relationship to another trying to fulfill her desires, and experiencing repeated disappointments.

In the Repertory, Platina is listed in italics under Ailments from Grief, but should probably be elevated to bold type, because the repeated griefs and disappointments in the love/sexual sphere lead to the fundamental Pathology of Platina. The Platina woman gives herself totally, and therefore experiences disappointments. As a consequence, on the mental plane, she ponders the issues of sexuality and love in the world, puzzling over the intensity of her needs. She is constantly seeking a way to balance her needs on both levels, but realistically, the world is unable to satisfy such excessive needs. She may then try to suppress the powerful sexual instinct into the mental plane, resulting in heightened idealistic, romanticized feelings. There occur a schism between the intense sexual desires and her highly idealistic beliefs. After many repeated emotional shocks and disappointments, there gradually evolves the process of PERVERSION of normal functions on these two levels.

On the mental/emotional level, one might expect such repeated griefs to lead to a bitter, vengeful, walled-off individual. In Platina, however, the particular perversion which occurs is a sense of exaggerated ego importance, of superiority, of haughtiness, of contempt for the world. The Platina patient feels she is more emotionally capable of love, that she has given herself more completely than other people. She feels that she is a unique individual, misunderstood by others with lesser capacities for love, not made for this world.

To summarise the process thus far, the Platina patient is driven at the outset by an exaggerated sexual desire and sensitive idealism, cannot be satisfied in the real world, experiences disappointment, s becomes tormented for along time by unsuccessful suppression into idealism, and eventually develops an exaggerated ego-sense and haughtiness.

In taking the case, the questioner may not be struck immediately by the haughty quality of the Platina patient. It will usually be difficult to recognise; one must read between the lines. In such a sensitive person, the suppression of sensuality into the mental sphere may result in a high degree of intellectualisation, or even spirituality. She may express her disappointments in the world, that there is not enough love and consideration in society. She may refuse to have children because it would be cruel to bring them into such a world (Ignatia, Natrum mur. and Staphysagria may also display such attitudes). The inner haughtiness may show as a contempt for the world, she may refuse to participate in dane conversations in company because of this attitude. At this stage of ego exaggeration, if recognised by the homoeopath, a dose of Platina will act quickly and easily, since the pathology has not yet advanced to a very extreme degree; treatment at later stages will also be successful, but may be longer and more arduous.

It is at this stage that the Platina patient may experience physical sensations or delusions which symbolise her internal conflict. Most characteristically, she feels as if parts of her body have enlarged in size, or that people and objects in the world have shrunk in size. Here is one vivid case example. A woman initially given Phosphorus, on a later visit finally revealed some peculiar symptoms; she would waken at night feeling as if she were in strange place, surrounded by strange furniture; the furniture seemed to float away, and people appeared small to her. In her own words, it was as if she were on a high hill looking at people far below her. Other remedies also have similar distortion; Sabadilla has the delusion that body parts are distorted, and Cannabis indica frequently has the delusion that the surroundings are distorted. In Platina, the delusion that parts of the body are enlarged may manifest instead as a feeling like bandage constricting the part, or there may be numbness of a part, particularly numbness around the lips, the area of the face most symbolic of sensuality. Also there may be a fear that the face is distorted, (and indeed, Platina is one of the remedies that can cure Bell's palsy).

Despite and haughtiness and contempt for the world which she experiences during the mental phase of her pathology, the Platina patient is at the same time driven by her powerful, earthy sexual desire. She is not really able to suppress it. So she will continue to be with men, but she may simultaneously maintain a feeling of contempt for them. Eventually, she may separate sex from romantic love, becoming interested in sex for the sake of

Platinum Metallicum

sensation only. Nymphomania then becomes increasingly evident in her behaviour. As the sexual urge becomes so intense that it cannot be satisfied, she will become increasingly involved in a variety of sexual perversions.

During the first stage of Platina pathology, the patient may alternate between the emotionally haughty state and intensely sexual state. While she is dominated more by her contemptuous, haughty behaviour, she will continue to be puzzled and intellectually preoccupied by the intensity of the earthy side of her nature. She may brood over this for a while, until the sensuality takes over and dominates her behaviour, resulting in nymphomania.

Alternations are common in Platina. As already mentioned, there may be an alternation between mental and sexual spheres. Mental symptoms and physical symptoms may also alternate; for example, the physical symptoms will disappear when the sensation of exaggerated size of a part of the body is present. As the delusion disappears, the physical symptoms return. Numbness of the face may alternate with fear of facial distortion.

In the second stage of development of Platina pathology, we see a given patient progressing in one of two directions of pathology. The direction of illness depends mostly upon the upbringing and background of the person. If she is in a culture in which her sensuality has been allowed free expression, her sexual nature will become more and more out of control. Perversions and nymphomania become increasingly manifest.

If she has actively controlled and repressed her desires, the previous mental defence represented by the inner contempt for the world becomes no longer successful. She may become snappish, sulky, sharp-tongued. There may be prolonged periods of brooding and depression. In desperation over the world's inability to satisfy her, she may even become suicidal, although she is unlikely to commit suicide. As the pathology progresses further, even depression no longer suffices, and she may experience a further perversion of her affection. She may feel a powerful desire to kill those closest to her, such as her husband and child (as is also found in Nux vomica, Mercury and even Arsenicum). In particular, this desire in Platina is stimulated by the presence or sight of a knife. This is a controlled desire to kill; Platina will rarely act on it. Such a desire, if purely unconscious, may manifest as an irrational fear that a fatal accident will befall her husband; she believes day in and day out that her husband will be killed, and she stays awake late into the night awaiting his return home.

In the third stage of Platina pathology, a true insanity develops, depending on which direction the pathology has taken. On the one hand, the haughtiness becomes exaggerated into an insane delusion of grandeur. Whereas previously she has kept such feelings largely to herself, in the insane stage it becomes overt. She believes she is royalty, that others are beneath her, that she is great and powerful and deserving of respect and deference. Unlike Veratrum album, who believes himself to be Jesus Christ or John the Baptist; an actual confusion of identity, and a sense of being given an important mission in life—the Platina delusion is an exaggerated sense of personal ego status.

The other form of Platina insanity manifests as an aggressive erotic mania. This is not merely the shamelessness or passive exposure of the genitals which we see in Hyoscyamus. It is practically indistinguishable from the erotic mania of Tarentula—an active, aggressive state, in which she will approach even strangers with an overt sexual proposition. The above-described essence of Platina is particularly evident in the physical symptoms. As mentioned there is the feeling of exaggerated size of parts of the body or of the entire body. This is also represented symbolically in the characterisitc Platina sensation as if a part is bound by a bandage (characteristic in an even stronger degree in Anacardium). There may be numbness (particularly around the lips), coldness, and cramping of muscles. There is a great hyperaesthesia of the genitals, becoming most painful to the touch, even to the point of preventing coition or speculum examination by the physician. Such hyperaesthesia seems to be caused by excessive congestion of the genitals and pelvic organs. *Platina* has even cured a pregnant woman who developed voluptuous spasms of the uterus, with orgasms which occurred so frequently and intensely that the spasms threatened spontaneous abortion.

To summarize then, the essence of Platina is a schism and perversion of the mental and sexual spheres, in a proud, sensitive woman, who has suffered repeated emotional disappointments, leading progressively to delusions of grandeur, or aggressive erotic mania.

PLUMBUM MATALLICUM (*plb.*)

The Plumbum patient is one which falls under the modern clinical category of ARTERIOSCLEROSIS. The Plumbum image is very similar to that seen in arteriosclerotic patients. It is a remedy which is very slow in its progression. The early pathology is barely noticeable but there is a slow and steady progression toward PARESIS on all levels.

Intellectually, there is a torpor, a sluggishness of mental functions. This slowness is seen both in perceptive and expressive functions. These patients are slow to receive impressions and slow to express themselves. This impairment is expressed quite dramtically by a characteristic symptom on the physical level—when stuck with a pin, they are a slow to react (this symptom is most striking in Cocculus, but is found in Alumina and Plumbum as well). There is slowness in perceiving external impressions, slowness of comprehension, and slowness in response.

A most characteristic impairment on the intellectual level in Plumbum is loss of memory—especially for words. This loss of memory in Plumbum is excessive in relation to the age of the patient. They strain to find the correct word for what they want to express, but they cannot. It is as if the specific location in the brain which governs this type of memory has had its circulation imparied by arteriosclerosis and has consequently atrophied.

Any intellecutal task is a great effort for Plumbum patients in full bloom. You ask a question, and they will be very slow to answer. This is not, however, the slowness of Phosphorus, which arises out of an emptiness in the head, nor is it the slow answering of Mercury, which is a result of confusion and distractibility. In Plumbum, the mind is sluggish in its functions, and the patient makes great efforts to answer your question. You see the knotted brow and the obvious effort involved in trying to come up with the answer. This is highly characteristic in Plumbum.

On the emotional level as well, there is a kind of paralysis which can best be described by the word APATHY. This is very similar to the stilled, apathetic state seen in old arteriosclerotic patients. There is no vitality, no movement of emotions inside. As is typical in Plumbum, this state does not come about overnight; it develops over a long period of time.

Plumbum pathology typically develops in "high livers"—people who have been egoistic and selfish throughout their lives. They have enjoyed the best of everything—the best food, the best surroundings, a model marriage etc. They become accustomed to these things, possessive about them. Eventually, they develop fixed "arteriosclerotic" attitudes and attachments. They eat rich foods, and they become easily upset over small things. These upsets stimulate the production of adrenaline in the bloodstream, which in turn increses the mobilisation of lipids. These then are deposited upon the linings of the arteries. Thus, selfish, possessiveness, and inflexible ideas lead to arteriosclerosis, which in turn leads to progressive panesis on all three levels of organism.

As these patients experience more and more apathy, they also become increasingly irritable and angry. In *Plumbum*, however, this irritability is characteristically expressed as an impulse to do harm to themselves. They become so nervous that they want to plunge a knife into themselves. This is a peversity, a desire to do self-destruction.

There is a sadness and gloominess in *Plumbum* which follows the stages of irritability. This is not a pure depression, but one which is coupled with anxiety. They seem to sense that their powers are waning, and consequently there is a fear that some calamity is going to befall them or their relatives.

Finally, the apathy gains the upper find. They hand no enjoyment in ordinary life. During the days of high living, they enjoyed sexual and other pleasures frequently. Once they become married, howerver, they find themselves impotent, again demonstrating the paretic state of *Plumbum*.

Interestingly, Plumbum patients counteract the apathy in a unique manner; they get involved in things which are unacceptable to society. They find excitement in risky, scandalous behaviour; they seek forbidden thrills. A married man may try to seduce his wife's sister, which, if discovered, would create incredible turmoil. In such a forbidden situation, he finds himself excited enough to regain his potency. Similarly, a married woman whose sister is married to a priest may have an affair with the priest. Plumbum may even be indicated in certain compulsive gamblers who gain thrills by risking their homes, businesses, etc., which are crucial to their very existence.

One may see an upright, church-going patient who suddenly decides to become a Buddihst, or to follow an Indian guru. Such behaviours create a tremendous turmoil among his family, friends, and colleagues. It is this upheaval which seems to counteract the apathy and paresis he has experienced. If his priest were to say,"O.K. go ahead", the patient would very likely lose interest in his new venture.

Plumbum patients have a distinct appearance which is dificult to describe. As mentioned, they have been accustomed to having the best of everything, so there is a kind of self-satisfied look about them. They tend to be skinny, and their faces have a somewhat earthy hue. There are deep lines in the face ,and deep pores:

Plumbum of course, is commonly indicated in patients suffering from neurogical problems. The Plumbum pathology is duplicated quite precisely by Parkinson's disease—whether of primary origin, or secondary to arteriosclerosis. The weakness, spasticity, trembling, and apathetic facial features are quite characteristic. *Plumbum* may also be indicated in patients who have had strokes, especially when there is paresis of extensor muscles. Both extensor and flexor muscles can be affected, but the most characterstic picture is extensor paralysis—such as we see in wrist-drop.

Plumbum patients experience trembling with the weakness of their muscles. It may be difficult for them to hold a glass steady. Spasms of the affected muscles are also quite typical. However, the spasms and twitchings are not as striking in *Plumbum* as they are in *Agaricus* and *Zinc*.

Specific groups of muscles may be the only ones affected, and atrophy of those muscles may be quite striking. When atrophy is a major aspect of a case, think of *Plumbum*. With this picture, it is easy to see that *Plumbum* should be prominent as a remedy in amyotrophic lateral sclerosis.

Plumbum paresis can affect the baldder and rectum as well. There may be retention of urine, even for as long as 24 hours. The urethral sphincter may become paralysed. Inactivity of the rectum may result in chronic constipation, with hard black stools.

Considering the arteriosclerotic tendency, it is not surprising the Plumbum fits a variety of circulatory disorders. Most characteristically, there is palpitation of the heart while lying on the left side—like *Lachesis* and *Phosphorus*.

Plumbum shares another keynote with *Phosphorus*—amelioration by rubbing. They have electric-like pains and cramps which are better from massage, most probably because the circulation is momentarily stimulated.

The most striking keynote of Plumbum is a drawing or pulling sensation in the umbilicus—as if a string is drawing the umbilicus toward the back. This sensation is not necessarily limited to the umbilicus; it can be felt anywhere in the abdomen, in the stomach, and even in the chest. This sensation is sometimes seen during a severe intestinal or renal colic, which is one circumstance in which Plumbum can produce results within a matter of hours.

Plumbum also has offensive foot sweat, like Silica.

According to Kent, *Plumbum* sometimes manifests as a hysterical state. I have not seen this myself, but the description given by Kent leads me to believe it. It has a condition similar to *Moschus*—the patient fakes illness. Kent quotes a case which stimulated comatose state in the presence of others, but was perfectly normal while alone.

Plumbum is a remedy which we do not see reported very frequently in the literature. I believe this is partly due to the fact that it is very slow in action. Many prescribers very likely do not have the patience to wait the many months required to see the full benefit of Plumbum; very likely its action is often disrupted by other prescriptions given too soon. In addition, Plumbum is most frequently indicated in elderly patients, in which the ultimate results are necessarily limited.

Alumina is one remedy which can appear somewhat similar to Plumbum. In Plumbum, however, the mental state is one of torpor, of flatness. In Alumina, there is a total confusion to the point of actual delusion—a chaos in which the patient is uncertain who is speaking. Also, the Plumbum paralysis does not reach the same severity as in Alumina. The Alumina paralysis is more

Plumbum Matallicum

of a flaccid paralysis, whereas Plumbum is more spastic; it is the difference between multiple sclerosis and Parkinson's disease. Finally the Alumina paralysis tends to affect the lower extremities, whereas Plumbum more commonly affects the hands and upper extremities.

PULSATILLA PRATENSIS (*puls.*)

Pulsatilla is primarily female. 75% of the time. Changeability with softness. A fluid yiedingness. No resistance to a challenge. May be slippery. Difficult to get symptoms. Very tuned in to what you want. (You must be careful to avoid any leading questions with a Pulsatilla patient). They shape themselves around whatever is presented with force. Strong feelings, but spontaneous. Not a strong sense of self-identity. Pulsatilla moulds herself to what others want. Phosphorus sees how others see her and buys that; Phosphorus is focussed on who she is because of her suggestibility. *Phosphorus* is suggestible, *Pulsatilla* is malleable. Pulsatilla is changeable, but basically simple, not complex. Pulsatilla is a river shaped by its surroundings. Phosphorus is a cloud, also changing, but diffusing. Phosphorus has strong imagination. Gullible. Sulphur has a big imagination which is very complex. Pulsatilla can not generalise about how she is because she changes. If someone says she is some way, she does not conjecture that it may be true, she tries to become that way. Sulphur is not changing; proud that he is into everything; always himself in all these things.

Pulsatilla's ideas are soft ideas. Not definite. Easily changed and shaped. Emotionally easily arousable. Quickly up for it if someone comes to her in a party mood. Physically, dischrges are changeable. No one pattern. Difficult to get modalities from her. Wandering symptoms. Menses changeable. Feminine, voluptous, large lips. Circulatory system easily relaxed and easily aroused. Easy flushing of face. Slow motion is characteristic. Gentle motion is most pleasant. Keeps her out of indolence, but exertion brings out her symptoms from the arousal. Ferrum becomes overexcited and overheated like Pulsatilla, but is tired and anaemic. Sensitive to noise, to the crinkling of paper. Not exciteable. Pulsatilla is aggravated by heat. Acute condition may he worse by cold. *Wilts* in a warm room. Worse by the sun. She can take the sun if she can walk or bathe frequently to cool off. Pulsatilla has sweltering heat. Phosphorus may have burning heat. Worse by warm drink (Like Phos.) Likes cold things. Not thirsty. Feet get hot.

Pulsatilla Pratensis

Must uncover them. Would not tolerate a sauna (Lachesis, Apis). Fear of closed places. Feels like she may suffocate. Ameliorated in cool water, sea shore etc. Intolerent to fat and food that makes her hot. Worse by alcohol, which over-stimulates her nervous system. Averse to fat, averse to pork. Craves or is averse to butter. Worse by changes (Nat. mur. which is closed off is worse in a closed room). Worse at twilight; morning person, wakes at dawn and loves the morning (Phos). Collapses at twilight (Phos). Phosphorus and Pulsatilla can be better at twilight.

Pulsatilla may be strong emotionally, if healthy and the symptoms are on the physical level. Weeps easily. Relieved by weeping. Pulsatilla is malleable, changeable. (Ignatia has internal conflict; idealistic, world fails them, they become cold and hard). Amelioration by consolation. May weep purposely in order to feel better. May get into a self-pitying state. She draws out your compassion. Relationships are very important. Needs a steadying, anchoring force. Forms a relationship, connects with someone, even a negative person as long as he is forceful. May be promiscuous early in life, but once a family is formed she is loyal.

Earth mother, loves to give and get massage. Sensuous. In a setting where culturally sensuousness is not accepted, she will suppress her desire and suffer from it. She will tell you that she misses it. High sexual desire; sexual physically and emotionally. Not so much through sexual fantasy. (Phosphorus loves the emotional contact, and high fantasy to sex, not so into the physical part.) A soft, well-spoken individual with nice tender feelings. Optimistic, but easily discouraged. Can never be aggressive or cruel. Does not want to impose. Sympathetic toward those close to her. May worry about a member of her family, but does not take on the other's feelings. A flower bending in the wind and looking for a stick to steady it. May become an extreme fanatic. Then she does not have to make a judgement of her own. Takes on someone else's attitude to the extreme. Food patterns may become rigid. Attracted to dogmas, to dogmatic, spiritual communities. Fickle, likely to change from one dogma to another. Can become so inflexible, she is nearly catatonic. Sits like a tree that needs to be watered. Apathy in end stage.

RHUS TOXICODENDRON (rhus-t.)

Stiffness, all over the body, especially on the joints. The jaw has stiffness and cracking. Emotional level is also incapable of spontaneous warmth, expression; some coldness. In love, they prefer the other shows love and affection to them, rather than they showing it. They have fear of being hurt. Become stiff in the mental level and get fixed iedas. Main idea—of being stiff and bound up, unable to relax. They feel tendons are stiff and hard, have to move all the time, stretching all the time to loosen them up. Very sensitive in the cervical region; stretching the neck all the time. Great sensitivity to draft on the cervical area—get a kind of dullness in the mind and then a kind of sleepiness. Worse in cold, damp weather. Will feel a draught, even if it is very minute (Kali carb.), but Kali carb. does not have the sensitivity in the cervical area. (Calc. phos., Cimic. are also sensitive in the cervical region). Worse after exposure to cold, wet and rain. Upper edges of trapezoid are mostly affected. Extreme restlessness, get relief from moving. First. movement is painful and relieving, but momentary and then they have to change positions again. He will be sitting there stretching, moving his legs, feeling as if a vice has caught the part that is stiff. When stiff, applying continuous effort to move. (Sepia has a kind of rhythm inside that has to be expressed through dancing). Stiffness and cracking in all joints, but mostly in the neck.

Irritated easily, not a big margin of tolerance (for aggravation, noises, etc.). Anxiety may progress into another state that is a fear that some bad misfortune will happen. Worse with weather changes; feel miserable, unhappy, discouraged and hopeless. Worse from water; for the Rhus tox, the water itself can eventually antidote the remedy. Better in warm, dry weather, locally and generally, relieves them emotionally as well. They themselves can't know warmth and emotion. Stiffness, bound up on the emotional level. Can get superstitious eventually, after fixed ideas on the mental plane. Worse evening when sun sets (Puls., Phos.). Can continue the whole evening through the night. Very much stiffness and pain at the moment he wakes up. Great desire for

Rhus Toxicodendron

milk. This may decrease after the remedy is given. Desire for cheese (Cist., Puls., Ign.). Desire for yoghurt (Nat sulph). Palsies, chorea, especially after exposure to wet or cold. Eruptions with vesicles, burning with great itching. Better with application of very hot water. Remedy that could be mistaken for Arsenicum, because of the restlessness, etc. Get fixed ideas that they might kill someone. (People suffering a lot with arthritis, on the mental/emotional level may not have too many symptoms or derangements).

SEPIA SUCCUS (*sep.*) (first version)

Stasis comes into mind when studying *Sepia*. Static which comes because of some action on dynamic plane. When the two poles of the energy in the body come together and cause a state of non-existence. (Naturally there is a bipolar condition in the body with the sex determined by a prevalence of one of the hormones in the body). What happens when hormonal balance is exactly the same in the body, is that a Sepia is produced. Exact balance of two opposing forces. (The urge for sex is the urge to bring about a balance, to release the excess of one or the other hormones). In Sepia, there is no need for such a release. Hormonal balance is equal, so are indifferent to sex. The idea of neutrality. Does not realise she has aversion to sex until the partner demands the sex, then she realises she has an aversion.

The idea of stasis. She does not have the natural curves of women. No curves, she is thin, flat-chested. (Ant. lobe of hypophysis is not working properly). If a woman has that build, the trouble is congenital. You will find it difficult to correct this balance. Sterility, inhabitual abortions (Miscarriages). Miscarriages are in the third to fifth month. Frigidity, great sensitivity in the hormonal balance. Stress can't be tolerated. Can be overthrown, out of balance, by having sexual intercourse quite frequently.

Idea of stasis on the physical level. Autonomic system has two opposing forces that clash and become neutralised. Statsis of uterus, prolapsus of uterus. Muscle becomes weak because of the loss of control by the autonomic nervous system. Sense of fullness in the rectum. She has constipation without urging. Empty feeling in the stomach, a kind of gnawing hunger. Aversion to food, even the smell. Constant nausea, worse in the morning (pregnancy morning sickness). Especially if there is an aversion to sex since she became pregnant. Aversion to husband. She eats and eats and can't get a full feeling. Vessels do not contract and dilate. Think of Reynaud's disease. Sepia has low blood pressure. A paralysis of the vessels; they are not functioning properly. White to red to blue, with the stasis, needs vigorous activity

Sepia Succus

to counteract. Better with vigorous activity. Walking fast and long. Emotional state also has same idea of stasis. Stillness of emotions. Feel without emotion. Can't be stimulated to have joy or emotion by any stimulus. The emotions that have been stilled refer to the affections. Affection and the joy of life. Can be so long in that state that she can't remember. Life is again running through her when she feels better. Anger, irritability, are easily produced in Sepia. She will hit the children in such a way. Does not feel the natural affection of a mother for her child. She is also unable to feel that natural affection or love for her husband. Logically, she can say he is nice, as long as she stays away from him in bed. When he makes demands then she will hate him.

Lumbago better with hard pressure. Palpitation on lying on the left side. Can't tolerate pressure around the neck (i.e. Lachesis). Tired, wants to stay alone; aversion to company. Can't eat fatty foods. This same picture with an aversion to sex makes it Sepia and not Lachesis. Fear she believes something can't be done. Sepia will usually cry during consultation. Spells of weeping. Brings all her suffering into the mind. Eventually she will develop tremendous anxiety, a feeling that something bad is going to happen. Sepia's anxiety is one of the worst. She will cry day and night and not know why.

Anxiety with an element of the unknown, that something is going to happen. This continuous weeping state must be after having been a Sepia for a long time. (Phosphoric acid will give a similar picture with the lack of feelings). In that emotional state, the best thing is to isolate herself. Nervousness, excitability in young girl with the skin. Laughing at a party; she will laugh, dancing. Tremendous excitability, in the children; as a little girl will have the impression that they can't break easily. Strained, excitable, flushing. Can't counteract the everyday stimulus in life.

The same stillness seems to prevail in the mind. Dullness; feels that she is stupid. Function of mental reflection is lost in her. The meaning of the question. Takes a long time for her to give the answer. Gets absent-minded. Indolence; aversion to do anything because she feels weak in her mind. Nothing seems to excite the dull, indolent mind. Stasis of the mind; no thinking going on. Better sitting with legs crossed. Prolapsus of the visceral organs. State of attachment. State of mind within its dullness can observe objectively because it is not involved. Sepia has no emotion—stillness of mind. She knows the weakness of everyone around her. That state of mind is similar to seekers of Truth; this idea of detachment, so deep inside has such a force; intellectual suppression, rather than submission. These seekers of Truth feel as if they cut down on emotion, forced detachment. They force on themselves a state of *Sepia*. Can have a guru in the state of *Sepia*. State where everything is so suppressed they can't come back to their normal life.

If you have a case spoiled by many remedies, Sepia is one that can bring back the case. You can suppress with drugs, or can suppress by will power. Male Sepia in comparison to female—one case to ten of female.

Stillness comes about by an intellectual process within the mind. Young man is sensitive and excitable. Once he is hurt, he tries to find an escape. To prevent this, he stills the emotions, and as much as is possible he controls the sex urge. Then comes an inability to think, a heaviness, dullness. Tries to activate the circulation of the body, and when he does this he feels better. Sepia has more of an aversion to salt.

SEPIA SUCCUS (*sep.*) (second version)

Chilly, better by vigorous motion (not exactly restless). Tall, thin, wiry (like models), pointed features, long fingers. Hard, caustic and harsh, perhaps competitive, hard driving. "The female Nux vom." Another Sepia is flabby, a little fat, beaten down, washer woman type, full of inertia, just can't do it any more. Swelling ankles, varicosities, prolapsed uterus, muscles flabby, collapses in a heap. A condition of stasis, stillness, stagnation, unresponsive to change. Inertia. A flaccid inertia. Relaxed, not tight. Baglike inertia. Requires a powerful stimulus to induce movement. A state of balance between maleness and femaleness. Female appears masculinised. Male appears feminine. Not reactive. No tension to create movement. Apathetic. Not interested in the opposite sex. Sympathetic and parasympathetic nervous system no longer dynamic, balanced state. No response. Uterus prolapses on standing, then gradually pulled back. Not the usual quick response, the change in gravitational force with change in position. Takes a great deal of stimulation to get a response. The balance is too equal. Needs stimulation to function. Static without stimulation. Takes any outside influence and makes a big deal out of it. Carried away, excitable by outside stimulation. Children very excitable (Phos). Sensationalism. Seeks anything that gets her going. Requires lots of stimulation in sexual functioning. Response to a sexual advance requires too much effort. Aversion to sex when approached. React with a feeling of repulsion through irritability, caustically. Frequent abortions, can't hold the foetus. Muscles flaccid. The essence of Ignatia is a highly charged lack of emotion. Ignatia is of two minds in balance, but in great conflict, resulting in tension and a steel-like hardness. Sepia is hard and cutting, sarcastic, penetrating. No sense of limits of how far she can go. Doesn't care if she hurts someone. Can be highly intelligent, penetrating mind. Sees through people and can remain unattached (pathological detachement). Not intentionally malicious. Senses that there is nothing moving inside. A deep secret that inside she really doesn't care. This frightens her, and causes her "causeless weeping". Feels there is no possible cure for her.

A fear that she is really not alive inside. Calc. has similar fear that there is no hope, tries to hide it. Both cry for similar reasons. Sepia can't explain why she is crying. Calc. also, because she feels she is going insane. Mind stills to an absence of thought (e.g. in middle age). Must do something to stimulate the mind to get it going; vigorous exercise, powerful stimulants, rubs forehead (Alum. to relieve the cobweb sensation, the veil over the mind.) Natrum mur. has a softness in the eyes; is physically similar to the thin early Sepia; romantic, but may lose her sexuality out of fear of rejection. It takes a lot to fill her stomach. It doesn't respond, doesn't feel full. May lash out against demanding children.

SILICA (*sil.*)

The key idea describing Silica patients is that they are YIELD-ING. It is a kind of shyness or timidity, but not really a cowardice (like Lycopodium or Gelsemium). It is a submissiveness that arises out of a lack of energy to insist upon his or her point of view, even though it may be strongly held. They are quite agreeable and mild, easy to get along with.

Silica patients are intellectuals, but not aggressive or critical like Lachesis. They have highly refined sensibilities, and they are very intelligent. If you try to impose an opinion upon a Silica person, she will not oppose you. She is sensitive to impressions and therefore takes into account your point of view. She understands very well where you are right and where you are wrong but she holds her opinions to herself. Unlike Pulsatilla, she has an opinion of her own, but she does not want to go to the trouble to impress it upon the world.

Thus, Silica appears mild and reserved—but not at all like Staphysagria, Ignatia, or Natrum mur. It is not an isolation. They are capable of freely talking about themselves when circumstances permit, and they make friends easily. They would never become dependent or demanding of the prescriber's time. For example, suppose you have been treating such a patient for some time without effect. The Silica patient will never challenge you or become impatient. She will not become dependent, like Arsenicum or Phosphorus. Silica does have the mildness of Phosphorus, but not the extroversion or dependency.

Silica patients are tired. They lack stamina, especially concerning mental work. Therefore, they learn to conserve their energies. They apply themselves to essentials, and they don't argue about irrelevancies—or merely in order to assert their ego.

Silica patients are very delicate, refined and aesthetic, even aristocratic. Consider for a moment what the term "refined" means; when something is refined, the coarse elements are removed from it. This is the case with Silica patients. They are thin, pale, delicate, and highly refined. They are intelligent and perceptive, but not assertive nor aggressive.

The classic Silica children come from elite, highly educated families. They are delicate, and they easily develop curvatures of the spine. Their intelligence is so great, however, that it has pathological consequences. It seems that they become over-stimulated, and then the lack of mental stamina results later in life. Most children, if corrected by their mother, will remember it for a few days and then go back to making the error. Silica children, however, never forget. They understand quickly the reason for the correction, and they impose upon themselves the correct behaviour. In a child, this represents excessive mental suppression. Silica children are too serious, too proper.

The overstimulation of mind followed by lack of stamina is the basis for the descriptions in the books of professionals who develop an aversion to their work. They feel incapable of performing their functions any more. This can be compared with Calc. carb., which may also have a lack of mental stamina, but this arises more from anxiety and worries. In general, Calcarea patients are more coarse, more survival-oriented. They worry about expenses, about unforeseen possibilities, etc. and they develop defences against these worries. Silica is more refined, delicate and vulnerable.

Just as Silica can be easily imposed upon, or suppressed, mentally, so this can occur on the physical plane. They tend to perspire profusely, especially in the axillae, the back of the neck, and on the feet, and they always do well as long as the perspiration is permitted. Do not be impatient to treat the Silica perspiration. If you succeed by any means in suppressing it, you and the patient will encounter a lot of trouble. If the sweat is suppressed by deodorants, foot powders, boric acid etc. the patient may well develop tuberculosis, cancer, kidney disease, or other serious disease.

Suppression of sweat by medication, of course, presents the most serious problems, but even evaporation can have similar effect—albeit less deep. If a perspiring Silica patient is exposed to a draft of air which evaporates the sweat, he may develop a headache or arthritic pains. The perspiration itself is highly characteristic in Silica. It is both offensive and acrid. The offensiveness is quite strong. The patient may wash his feet three times a day

Silica

to no avail. The odour arises from the discharge of toxins—like *Psorinum*, but not nearly so severe; it is impossible to even remain in the same room with a Psorinum patient. *Sulphur*, of course, is famous for offensive perspiration, but this arises from inadequate washing. Sulphur patients, lost in their minds, wash only in spots and not very thoroughly—a symptom which, of course, is difficult to elicit except by direct (and diplomatic) questioning.

The Silica foot sweat is also acrid. This is not a merely irritating perspiration; it actually chews up socks. If a normal person uses up a pair of socks every two years, the Silica patient uses them up within three months.

Considering the reserved, submissive mental state of Silica patients, it is not surprising that they develop tumours of all kinds—fibromas, breast cysts, swollen glands, warts etc. These tumours are usually hard, (like Calc. fluor, and Baryta mur). They even develop keloids, like Graphites. Fissures are another common skin complaint. The nails are brittle, and most characteristically, they have many white spots on the nails.

Of course, Silica is famous for opening up deep abscesses, and curing patients who have a tendency to suppurations. This is true when it fits the patient as a whole. Because Silica is a very deep-acting remedy, it is risky practice to routinely prescribe it whenever an abscess needs opening. In patients with suppurative tendencies, Silica may help in the moment, even when it does not fit the patient as a whole. What effect will it have for the suppurations which will develop later—which may well be rendered more deep and more resistant to treatment?

The submissiveness of *Silica* displays itself characteristically in regard to its well-known constipation. The stool is hard, and the rectal muscles are inactive. There is great straining, but the stool slips back inside, and the patient gives up. The books appropriately, call it "bashful stool".

Considering the food tendencies Silica has an aversion to salt, meat, and milk. There is an intolerance to both fat and milk. I have also observed that Silica can have a desire for eggs (like Calc. carb. and Pulsatilla).

If you encounter a patient with very little mental or emotional symptomatology it can be somewhat difficult to differentiate Silica from Nitric acid. Both tend to be thin and chilly. Both have acrid perspiration. Both have tumours, warts and fissures. Both have white spots on the nails. On purely physical symptomatology, the key differentials are salt and fat. Nitric acid desires fat and salt, whereas Silica is averse to salt and intolerant to fat. Of course, usually the emotional symptoms make the differentiation unmistakeable. Nitric acid is very anxious, dependent, and demanding. Silica on the other hand, is more considerate, patient, and yielding.

Silica feels the cold strongly, but one must also remember that, during acute ailments, Silica can also be intolerant to warm stuffy rooms—like *Pulsatilla.* Conversely. Silica can be aggravated by drafts, even though he or she may not feel the draft particularly. This is in contrast to *Kali carb.*, which feels the draught but is not much aggravated by it. Sometimes, Silica is ameliorated when the weather turns to dry cold.

It is very interesting that *Silica*, like *Calcarea* is aggravated during full moon. It seems that patients which are lacking in elements which are prevalent in the earth—and probably the moon as well—are affected by moon phases.

Silica patients have a peculiar relationship to pins. They do not volunteer this fact, but you can elicit through questioning that they have a fear of pins and of pointed things. This can occasionally be useful confirmatory symptom. Another peculiar Silica symptom is the sensation of a hair on the tongue—like *Kali bich.*

Silica patients do not usually develop severe pathology on the emotional or mental planes, in my experience. They mostly complain of a lack of mental stamina. Sometimes they may develop fixed ideas, which is not surprising in view of the formation of hard tumours. They have absolute prejudices which they simply cannot alter; i.e. "Sex is sinful under any circumstances." It is as if a small portion of the brain has become sclerosed, causing a loss of flexibility in thinking in regard to specific concepts.

STANNUM METALLICUM (*stann.*)

The word which characterises *Stannum* is EXHAUSTION. Whenever a patient presents as a main complaint general debility, on whatever level, *Stannum* is one of the main remedies to keep in mind. There is a deep and chronic weakness and debility which colours every aspect of the case.

The Stannum appearance is quite distinctive. These are old tuberculous patients—people who had tuberculosis 20 years ago and now they complain of colds, flu, and many bronchial problems. Throughout their lives, they become progressively weak until each cold leads to great exhaustion and bronchial troubles with copious, sweet-tasting mucous; the bronchi are a clear region of localisation with *Stannum*. These people have skin which is yellowish-copper in colour. The skin has a thickness to it—like leather. Stannum people are skinny, exhausted and pale. You will never see a Stannum patient with a rosy colour such as you see in Pulsatilla, Ferrum, or Calc. carb.

The exhaustion of Stannum is almost without parallel. The weakness is so great that they have a feeling of heat under the skin. They even say that their eyes are "burning from weakness". Another description they use is that the weakness seems to be felt flowing through the veins. Fatigue, of course, is a fairly common symptom in sick patients, but in Stannum it is so striking that the patients use such vivid imagery to describe their feelings.

The exhaustion in Stannum is so great that even the slightest exertion becomes a great source of aggravation. They become exhausted even from the effort of talking; whenever a patient tells you that he becomes short of breath after talking for a few minutes on the phone, be sure to think of Stannum. To observe such a patient sitting quietly in chair, you would never imagine the severity of his condition. However, if you ask the patient to go over to the examination table, he immediately becomes so short of breath that you become alarmed. Even the act of going to the basin to wash his face in the morning is a great effort. In my experience, there is only one other remedy which has such great exhaustion, Helonias; in Helonias the very act of rising from a chair causes great flushing and exhaustion.

Some Stannum patients may not yet have reached such an extreme degree of exhaustion, but in any case fatigue and weakness will be the leading symptom in every Stannum case. Even if he is able to continue working, he is exhausted by his usual standards and takes every opportunity to lie down.

Such extreme aggravation from exertion naturally makes one think of *Bryonia*, but there is a great deal more animation in Bryonia than in Stannum. Even in a Bryonia patient going toward coma, there still will be a lot of irritability. He may seem to be on his last legs, but if you go near him, he will react. Stanum is far more exhausted than that. He feels so weak that he is certain he is going to die within a few years.

Stannum patients do not actually fear death. They feel so weak that they rationally feel that death is near. They naturally feel a despondency and discouragement. At first they develop an anxiety about the future. They wonder, "How am I going to live? What am I going to do?" This is an appropriate anxiety, of course, even though it may be carried a bit to an extreme.

Finally, they seem to give up the fight against the disease. They do not have the energy to do anything but despair. This is not an anxious despair, like Calc. carb. or Arsenicum. It is a true despair.

Because of the tremendous exhaustion, Stannum patients do not want to see people. It is not that they do not like people; indeed, Stannum people are very sweet, undemanding individuals who get along well with people—somewhat like Silica. They are simply too exhausted to cope with the exertion of greeting someone. The books describe this symptom as a "dread" of people, but it is not nearly so strong or fearful a state as dread. It is simply a tremendous exhaustion that renders conversation impossible.

Sometimes Stannum patients get into a kind of hysterical state in which they are easily distractable and inefficient. They begin one task, then get off into another and the another—without getting anything done. A woman may begin doing a particular calculation, then she suddenly recalls that she has to prepare the tea for her husband, then the trash must be taken outside etc. It seems that the

Stannum Metallicum

weakness of the mind becomes so great that it cannot maintain its focus. Other ideas intrude, and the patient cannot set them aside or organise them properly.

These exhausted, tubercular patients experience neuralgias which gradually build up and then gradually decrease. Typically, Stannum symptoms increase and decrease during daytime hours—following the sun, as it is described in the books. This is not truly an aggravation from exposure to the sun; rather, it is a gradual crescendo which begins around mid-morning, peaks around 2 p.m., and then a decrescendo by late afternoon. Stannum headaches, for example, are typically worse between 10 a.m. and 4 p.m. This approximates the 10 a.m. to 3 p.m. aggravation of Natrum mur., but extends later in the afternoon and has a typical rising and falling curve of intensity.

Also Stannum complaints—whether neuralgia, headache, cough, or lumbago—have a characteristic 5 a.m. aggravation.

Stannum patients often describe a characteristic weakness in the chest, even if they do not suffer from the usual tuberculosis, dyspnoea, or bronchial asthma. It seems to be a kind of emptiness, but patients usually use the term "weakness". It especially comes on while the patient is talking. I have seen this many times in Stannum.

There is a peculiar symptom in Stannum; anxiety before menses, ameliorated with the flow. This is a strong characteristic. Such a symptom would suggest *Lachesis*, but be sure to remember *Stannum*, especially in a patient complaining of fatigue, extreme aggravation from slightest exertion, and daytime aggravation.

Phosphoric acid of course, is a remedy which is often thought of in exhausted patients, but this is much more of an emotional weakness. The main characteristic of Phosphoric acid is apathy. A Phosphoric acid patient can watch his house burn down, and he won't feel moved at all. Stannum patients, however, do have feelings in spite of their exhaustion. A young Stannum girl with tuberculosis can fall in love with a man; she has feelings. A Stannum man can enjoy his new car, where as Phosphoric acid patient would be completely indifferent about such a thing.

Muriatic acid is another remedy which has tremendous debility, but he is not conscious of it. Like Opium, the Muriatic acid patient incorrectly feels that nothing is wrong. Usually, the Muriatic acid weakness applies more to acute situations—a fever and septicaemia that bring about complete exhaustion, especially on the physical level. This, however, is a completely different situation and is not easily confused with Stannum.

STAPHYSAGRIA (*staph.*)

The main idea characterising *Staphysagria* is SUPPRESSION OF EMOTIONS, particularly those centering around romantic relationships. Staphysagria patients are very excitable, very easily aroused. Their problems are then compounded when they do not allow natural outlets for their arousal. It can manifest in basically two ways which are typified by women and men. In women, the emotional suppression results in a state of sweet passivity and resignation—a kind of timidity. In men, this sensitivity may not be so obvious; to the outside world they may appear masculine, even hard, but inside they experience the same kind of delicate sensitivity and romantic vulnerability.

The Staphysagria woman is rather delicate and highly strung. She is a nice person, very considerate of others. She is a person who feels her problems belong to her alone. She would never presume to be a burden to others. At the outset of the homoeopathic interview, the Staphysagria patient offers very little information. She tends to talk only about the specific problems. It is not that she is a closed person in the true sense; she is merely reluctant to become burdensome to the prescriber. The Staphysagria woman is not outgoing or forceful. She is reserved, but with a sweetness. If the prescriber shows sincere interest and sympathy, the patient will open up quickly. This is in marked contrast to Ignatia, which is truly reserved; the Ignatia patient is aloof and guarded—difficult to open up.

The Staphysagria patient is never egoistical, harsh, or proud. Even the Staphysagria man, who may appear strong and masculine to outward appearances, is very sensitive and timid inside. There is a true humility arising from an internal assumption of powerlessness. The Staphysagria patient feels unable to fight even for her own rights. In early years, she experiences a few confrontations—however minor—and quickly learns to submit to any quarrel or imposition.

Even when she is in the right—when someone treats her unjustly—she will not fight back. She swallows her indignation, but the key distinction in Staphysagria is that there is no bitterness. The passive suppression of emotions is then the trigger for the pathological picture of Staphysagria. Although she remains sweet in her sense of powerlessness there is a deep weakening of the healing process internally. A kind of hardening or INDURATION develops on the mental plane. The emotional wound never quite heals, and the patient's innate sensitivity increases to an even greater degree. She feels even more vulnerable, less assertive, and consequently suppresses her emotions even more than previously.

The process of induration as a result of suppression is particularly visible on the physical plane. Wounds do not heal easily. It is not that they fester or become "bitter", to carry further the analogy from the emotional plane. Instead, the damaged tissues become hardened and indurated. There is the development of hard, dead tumours, or chronic indurations of various kinds. This is particularly true in relation to sexual organs (ovaries, uterus, testes)—as one might expect considering the romantic/sexual arousal and sensitivity in the Staphysagria patient. A good example of this process is found in the evolution of styes. In Staphysagria, styes not only come and go as in other people, but they leave small hardened spots of induration which do not go away with time.

Staphysagria is one of several remedies which are characterised by ailments from grief. Again, in Staphysagria there is a kind of "sweetness" in the face of grief. By contrast, Ignatia and Natrum mur. patients who have experienced many griefs become bitter; it is as if there is a thorn inside, and they become hard to reach. If you probe deeply in such patients, you see a bitterness, a harshness, which is prickly like a thorn. In Staphysagria, on the other hand, your probings encounter a kind of sweet resignation.

A key aspect of the Staphysagria ailments from grief is that they are always in regard to romantic relationships. The long term suffering they experience rarely arises out of such griefs as professional setbacks, financial reversals, or even deaths in the family. They are nice people, and they get along well with people; if there is an occupational reversal, they recover easily and move on. By contrast, Aurum patients collapse totally after a business failure; they suffer a loss and shoot themselves or jump from a high building. In Ignatia or Natrum mur., a careful past history will reveal the onset of problems after deaths of relatives or loved ones. In Staphysagria, the suffering occurs more commonly in regard to romantic disappointments.

The Staphysagria patient's sweet resignation is a kind of timidity, even though Kent does not list Staphysagria in the rubric Timidity. The reason for this is that such patients may not appear timid in public, in their occupations, at parties etc. They are nice people and they can be quite friendly. Their timidity occurs whenever they meet someone to whom they feel romantically attracted. Then they develop an active fantasy life, but they fear too much closeness; this is the origin and setting for their timidity.

The Staphysagria patient, as I have said, is highly excitable. He or she is easily aroused in a romantic relationship. The mental realm of fantasies and romantic imagery is greatly stimulated. She thinks about her lover all day long. Before falling asleep at night, she replays in her mind past encounters with her lover and imagines future possibilities. Her problem arises, however, when the relationship comes to the reality. She is more comfortable at a distance. She can be easily and fully satisfied by a purely platonic relationship. Such a patient can derive great pleasure from such a mental relationship for many years.

Because of her high degree of arousal and the fact that no natural outlets are allowed for her feelings, the Staphysagria patient places too much importance on little things. Small gestures, whether her lover greets her with the expected enthusiasm, etc. become exaggerated out of all proportion to reality. She can be easily satisfied by small things, but she may also suffer great agony over them. For this reason—and also because of her reluctance to proceed beyond the realm of mentalised romanticism—many of her relationships fail to last. She experiences disappointments, and her vulnerability increases.

Thus, in Staphysagria patients you see many romantic griefs. They become easily aroused, fantasize, and then are disappointed. It is after repeated such episodes that they develop pathology on the physical level. After a disappointment—or a confrontation—they suffer diarrhoea, frequent urination, the development of hardened tumours, enlarged prostate, etc. They may suffer from headaches, especially a peculiar wood-like sensation in either frontal or occipital regions. This sensation of wood is highly characteristic, and it corresponds to the process of induration found on other levels as well.

It is important to emphasise that Staphysagria patients are very easily excited. All five senses can be aroused to fever pitch. This, coupled with their fear of intimacy, naturally leads to the strong tendency toward masturbation for which Staphysagria is famous. The Staphysagria patient's fantasy reaches such a great intensity that it demands an outlet, so the patient satisfies this demand by masturbation.

Because of their high degree of sensitivity, Staphysagria patients are often artisically inclined. This inclination, however, usually involves solitary artistic activities—painting, music, poetry. It would be very ususual to find Staphysagria indicated in an extroverted stage actor or singer. You may encounter, for instance, a sea captain requiring Staphysagria. Your first impression would never suggest Staphysgaria for a man in a position requiring such assertiveness and hardness. But then you discover that internally he has a quite refined aesthetic sense; he spends his leisure hours writing romantic poetry. Such an image could lead to Staphysagria.

I remember a 35 year old man who responded very well to Staphysagria. He was a nice man, he made friends easily, but he had a chronic reluctance to becoming involved in a real love affair. It was not that he was homosexual; he merely feared intimacy. He admitted to me that his major problem was masturbation. He felt compelled to masturbate daily from the age of 7 to the age of 35. At some level he felt that this was excessive, and he repeatedly resolved to control himself; but by the next day his will was weak, and he continued his habit. This had become a tremendous problem for him. I believe, if he had not received Staphysagria, he would eventually have degenerated into a terrible condition.

Such sensitive people, when they experience griefs or direct confrontations, are strongly affected in the nervous system in particular. They immediately suffer internal trembling, and this may eventually evolve into outright chorea. The circulatory system may also be affected; there may occur high blood pressure or unequal distribution of blood in the body. The face may be red

Staphysagria

or white, and the lips may be blue.

From the image presented so far, the reader can easily predict the effects of *Staphysagria* on the sexual sphere. At first there is great arousal, particularly when not actually in the presence of the lover. This arousal is released through masturbation. But whenever confronted with an actual sexual situation, the patient becomes impotent or frigid.

In children, of course, we do not see the same image as in adults. Nevertheless suppression is still the major theme. You may see mental retardation caused by suppression of natural inclinations brought about by parents or teachers. I recall a case of an 11 year old child who had been intelligent, friendly and outgoing until he went to school at the age of 6. By his second year in school he was already falling behind in his work. By the time he saw me, he appeared to everyone to be mentally retarded. He had completely missed 3 full years of school. His behaviour was very troublesome. He used to strike his mother so much that at first I prescribed Stramonium, without effect. Finally, I realised that the turning point in this case occurred when he entered school, so I probed persistently about the circumstances around that time. It turned out that the mother and father used to fight a great deal, which undoubtedly affected the child, but this had been true over a period of years. Finally, I discovered that he had been left-handed by nature, until the teacher forced him to write with the right hand "like all the other children." From past experience I knew that such a suppression could be a powerful influence. On this basis, I gave Staphysagria and this child is now not only able to keep up with is schoolwork, but he is rapidly making up the 3 years he had lost.

In later stages of Staphysagria pathology, the over sensitivity can manifest as excessive irritability. Staphysagria can become destructive and violent—not as much as Stramonium, but to a significant degree nevertheless. In this stage, one can easily mistake *Staphysagria* and *Coffea*. Both are very excitable. Their senses, especially hearing, can become very sensitive; although not comparable with Stramonium.

The stages on the mental level are quite predictable from the basic Staphysagria image. At first, after a strong grief or confrontation, there is internal trembling. Later, this may develop into chorea; I have seen several cases of chorea cured by *Staphysagria*. Next, one may see loss of memory. The patient becomes mentally fatigued and forgetful. He or she may read something and cannot remember what has just been read. The induration which is so prominent on the physical level eventually reaches into the mental level as well. The intellect becomes "indurated", inflexible. A kind of dementia develops. The patient cannot properly receive new ideas or external impressions, and he or she just sits and stares. Again, along with many other remedies, Staphysagria can be indicated in senility when the previous history shows a process of chronic suppression and induration.

EXTRA NOTES! Sex may degenerate into lasciviousness or lustfulness. An enjoyment beyond what is natural. Overindulging into sex relationships. Finds himself in a state where everyone dictates what he is doing with them (if in a lot of relationships). May create in his mind a state where he has no reigns on his life; everyone can do whatever they like. Let themselves get into situations that they did not really approve of. Cannot say no. So, a mess may develop after a while. Enlargement of the prostate gland can come about because of promiscuity, lustfulness, or maintaining long erections to satisfy others. So, forces the hormonal system to work in an unnatural way. Impotent after all the previous exertions—corrected by Staphysagria (with Lycopodium being the main remedy for impotency). May have painful erections in the night, out of the blue, long-lasting ones that are very painful.

STRAMONIUM (*stram.*)

As described by Kent, the first thing which impressed one about Stramonium is the violence of the mental state. It is a very active, agitated, driven state. The person is out of control, destructive, even malicious in behaviour. It is destructiveness of all kinds—against other persons or oneself, striking, biting, tearing, shrieking, cursing—but most expecially, smashing things. Such a state may erupt rather suddenly, then subside after a while, but the person is not free of it. Typically, it is a chronic mania, or relapsing frequently over a period of time, rather than just a simple paroxysm of rage.

The primary process in the Stramonium state is an uncontrolled eruption of the unconscious, leading to violent, aggressive behaviour. In the normal sane person, the contents of the unconscious—evolutionarily, the animal instinctual level—are kept under tight control by the higher cerebral functions, the conscience, societal and cultural influences, and moral and religious values. When a person becomes insane, almost by definition these controls are loosened, or distorted, so that behaviour deviates from the norm. In the Stramonium state, the unconscious instincts erupt with awesome suddenness and violence and there appears to be no chance for the normal mechanisms to establish any degree of control.

This type of insanity is seen in the most extreme cases. It might be indicated in a mass killer who suddenly begins killing many people indiscriminately; of course, one would never prescribe SOLELY on such an indication (another possible remedy might be Nux vomica for example) but *Stramonium* would have to be at least THOUGHT of in such a case. One would think of Stramonium in the type of mental patient in whom there is no choice except forcible restraint in a padded cell.

One limitation of the Repertory is that it does not indicate the STAGES of development of symptoms. Thus, while many remedies are listed in the rubric Violent, one has no way to discover at what stage the violence becomes evident. In Stramonium although the onset of the violent stage may be fairly sudden, there are discernible stages prior to it. Their recognition is very useful in deciding on the prescription.

The original cause of the Stramonium insanity is a sudden shock. There may be a sever fright, an emotional shock, a head injury, or a fever affecting the brain (if the latter, it is quite likely that there will be spasms or convulsions at even a relatively low level of fever). The emergence of the unconscious then begins to show its appearance by symptoms such as extreme fear of the dark—they need the light on all night. There may be unusual fears such as a fear of cemeteries, (Stramonium is commonly found growing in cemeteries), a fear of tunnels or closed places, fear of even viewing a large body of water, fear of dogs. Particular symptoms may be triggered at night in the dark—there is a definite aggravation from darkness—or upon viewing the surface of a body of water. In the books it is said that *Stramonium* is aggravated by glittering objects such as shining metal, mirrors, fires; from experience, however, this is more commonly seen in relation to the surface of a body of water. Symbolically, such symptoms represent early signs of the eruption of the unconscious, barely controlled. Next, there may be spasms in various parts of the body—the eyes, the neck, the limbs.

The culminating stage is a full-blown eruption of the unconscious into violent insanity. You may get a telephone call from a relative that the patient has suddenly begun smashing windows and furniture and threatening to kill family members. This is the type of patient who would need immediate hospitalisation, restraints, and sedatives in the orthodox approach. When you see the patient, he is aggressive and out of control, or he sits in a chair with a rigid posture and a wild look in his eyes, anxious wrinkles on the forehead, about to jump up and run out of the house at any moment.

On questioning, you discover that he has been urgently insisting that the light be left on at night, and anxiously desiring company at all times. Perhaps he has been staying awake at night weeping, then laughing immoderately during daytime hours.

If left untreated, such a case would inevitably be institutionalised and restrained. With time, the mental state may degenerate into a convulsive disorder, or the common syndromes of organic

Stramonium

brain syndrome or senility.

There is a relationship to rabies, or hydrophobia—Stramonium will sometimes cure such cases. The hydrophobic state is also triggered by water, either seeing or hearing water. There is a strong aversion to drinking water also.

Stramonium has a striking delusion of being attacked by dogs, A FEAR OF DOGS that might attack.

The acute stage of Stramonium may be compared with Belladonna. There may be a high fever of sudden onset, particularly caused by meningo-encephalitis. In Stramonium, the fever may or may not be as high as in Belladonna, but the Stramonium fever is relapsing or continuous, in contrast with the remittent Belladonna. One may reasonably give Belladonna with the first episode; if the fever returns, however, Belladonna will no longer be of value. One must turn to other remedies; if there is violent, aggressive delirium, with the usual Belladonna picture of flushed face, dilated pupils, dry mouth, spasms etc., then Stramonium should at least be considered. The Stramonium delirium is as described above—smashing things, biting, tearing clothes, shrieking, cursing. He is unaware of his surroundings, of other people, and even of his own sufferings. In his activity he may display superhuman strength (Tarentula). The child in the office sits rigidly clutching the chair in fear, staring with a wild look in the eye, ready to pounce or run. When the acute mania subsides the patient falls into the alternate state of anxiety and despair.

One needs to be aware in studying remedies of where the focus of action resides. In *Stramonium* the focus has to do with the unconscious, perhaps even specifically the rage centre in the hypothalamus. There is a clinical syndrome known to neurologists having to do with head injuries causing a basal skull fracture and damage to the hypothalamus, resulting in specifically the type of rage and disorientation described in Stramonium. A similar picture can occur in severe extremes of alcoholic intoxication, when the person loses all control and flies into an irrational rage.

Stramonium also powerfully affects the peripheral nervous system. Particularly it produces a spastic state of the neuromuscular system. It has benefited considerably spastic children afflicted by birth injury or neonatal jaundice. It can relieve the spastic kind of paralysis seen in stroke victims and other neurological damage.

It also has the graceful, rhythmic, involuntary motions of chorea—particularly affecting the upper extremities. Again, the emphasis is on involuntary, uncontrolled conditions of the nervous system.

Although relatively less striking, *Stramonium* does have some effects on the physical level. Some highlights; headaches which are aggravated by sun, worse from heat, worse from lying and worse from motion, located usually in the occiput but also may be in the forehead. Basilar meningitis from suppressed otitis media. Strain of the eyes from prolonged studying. Strabismus if caused by brain fever or injury. Chronic abcesses, boils, and septic states, particularly when accompanied by spasms and convulsions. It has severe pain in the left hip (bold type in the Repertory). A peculiar cough triggered by looking into a bright light or into a fire. A sense of suffocation when water is poured on his head. In old men, retention of the urine due to spasm of the bladder.

So, in comparison with the other remedies, the point to emphasise is the malicious, violent, aggressive, uncontrolled eruption of the unconscious, particularly in chronic and sustained manias. *Stramonium* is the most violent, then *Belladonna* and finally *Hyoscyamus*. The Belladonna violence is mostly in acute states. During the *Belladonna* delirium we see that the patient wants to climb up the walls of the room. He gets up from bed, with a very high fever, and you see him struggling to climb up the walls in a wild state. The delusions of Belladonna also should be stressed, especially on closing the eyes. Striking at people is also a strong symptom of *Belladonna*. Hyoscyamus is more passive in its mania, being violent when moved by extreme jealousy or when pushed to an extreme. Desire to strike is a strong symptom of *Hyoscyamus*. The rage in Tarentula occurs more in paroxysms. The Veratrum state is as active and energetic as Stramonium, but not usually as violent except in extreme circumstances.

SYPHILINUM (*syph.*)

- Fear about everything < lying down.
- Anxiety +++
- In evening all anxieties go away and feel calm.
- Perspire with slightest emotion. Perspire even sewing a button.
- Fear of catching cold—so strong will stay indoors.
- Anxious enquiry—convinced something can be done for them.
- Loss of self-confidence—don't know if what they do is right or wrong.
- Check things 10 times over. (Phos., Caust.)
- Different kinds of fear—not knowing what afraid of.
- Develop a tremendous aversion to anything dirty after sex with a prostitute. May become so strong will wash clothes if someone touches them in a bus. Will not even shake hands with you. Wash hands 50—200 times daily—shrivelled skin on hands.
- Successful being one-pointed in their profession—become very meticulous and very proficent.
- If not able to wash hands will develop sweat, headache.
- Paranoid fear that if their children touch what they have touched they will be similarly tainted. Know this is ridiculous but do not have strength to stop.
- Will ask, "Do you think I am going crazy?"—until you give them the answer they want, which is no.
- < night.
- Sleepless. Wake 2—3 a.m. cannot get off again.
- Superstition—if throw something away create a bad fate for themselves, think something will happen.
- Anxiety about health—but they will deny it.
- Anxious about winter—so cold, how shall I move about?
- If a cat passes near clothes when on washing line, has to wash them again.

Works best in very high potency—50 M, CM. Don't expect it work quickly. May have to wait six months—a year for any action to develop. (Silica also slow to act).

Suppressed syphilis will produce alcoholism, also a super-ego. *Causticum* is more direct, and if wakes and thinks has left door open will get up immediately to close it. *Syphilinum* will lie and think something is going to happen before getting up to check it.

TARENTULA HISPANICA (*tarent.*)

Tarentula hispanica, although it has many symptoms in common with other remedies mentioned, it also has a particularly distinctive personality.

The primary focus of action of *Tarentula*, especially in the first stages, is on the nervous system. The nervous system in Tarentula seems wound up tight like a coiled spring, tense with boundless energy which must be expended to prevent it from breaking. The Tarentula patient is compelled to be busy, to act, to move constantly without ceasing. The early stages may be found most characteristically in people in occupations requiring much detailed work while under great pressure and responsibility, such as air traffic controllers or news journalists confronted with deadlines. The constant pressures result in a keyed up, oversensitive nervous system. Like *Nux vomica*, the Tarentula patient may initially be a compulsive worker. Such people seem to have super-human stamina, capable of and even compelled to work day and night, perhaps without sleep for weeks on end. They are industrious, capable, efficient; but unlike Nux vomica which is driven by a mental ambition and competitiveness, the Tarentula patient is driven by the nervous tension, the sheer compulsion to move and to keep busy.

Tarentula is—along with Sulphuric acid—the most hurried of all the remedies listed in the Repertory; many are listed in this rubric in strong grades, but Tarentula and Sulphuric acid lead them all. There is constant restlessness, most particularly of the lower extremities, but also of the entire body. Other remedies are characterised by such restlessness, but not to the extreme degree of Tarentula. The Tarentula patient will spend the whole night tossing and turning in bed until he finds himself with his head at the foot of the bed and the sheets tied in knots.

The *Tarentula* restlessness and nervous tension affects primarily the nervous system from the cerebellum and downward into the spine. Reading the Materia Medicas, the collection of symptoms belonging to it seem often inseparable from *Arsenicum*, but the

Arsenicum restlessness arises from the mental/emotional plane, and it never has the excessive energy of *Tarentula*; it is an anxious anguished restlessness which only secondarily causes the characteristic restless changing of positions. Veratrum is also very hyperactive, but from an overactive mind. In Tarentula, the restlessness arises out of a need to release extreme nervous energy, which results in anxiety and activity of the mind as secondary effects to the disturbance in the nervous system itself.

The Tarentula activity is always very fast. Everything must be done with the greatest speed. He is even impatient with slowness in other people; if someone is walking slowly on the street, the Tarentula patient may become angry and urge the person to move along more quickly. On his way home, the Tarentula patient may walk faster and faster, until finally he is actually running the last leg. This arises not so much out of a sense of anticipation but out of a compulsion for sheer rapid motion.

Because of the wound-up state of the nervous system, the Tarentula patient is relieved by rhythmic activities and influences. Particularly striking is the soothing and calming influence of the rhythmic vibrations of music. Rhythym seems to channel and release the tension, thereby calming and quieting the nervous system. This is a different mechanism from the improvement from music seen in Aurum, which soothes more directly the mental level, or in Natrum mur. in which music produces a relaxing harmonious environment. Of course, the wrong type of music, particularly at a time when the Tarentula patient is under great pressure, can also trigger off and aggravate the wound-up state. The need for rhythm is the reason for the tendency of Tarentula patients to dance, to jump, and to run; and these movements are not merely gentle and slow. Tarentula patients are driven to wild, frenzied, rapid and vigorous movements. At the same time, however, the movements are graceful, rhythmic and flowing; thus *Tarentual* is a prime remedy to consider in choreas, such as St. Vitus' Dance of Huntington's Chorea.

Such a wound-up nervous system is not surprisingly affected by external pressures and influences. As mentioned, music of the wrong type may aggravate the condition. For the same reasons, Tarentula patients are markedly aggravated by touch. A striking feature is aggravation from bright or strong colours—red, yellow, green, black.

There is a lot of anxiety in *Tarentula*, anxiety that things will not get done, that something will go wrong. It is often an irrational fear, but it is a fear that again arises out of the wound-up state of the nervous system. On the other hand, the Arsenicum anxiety is a primary state on the emotional plane itself.

In the first stage, *Tarentula* is also a hysterical remedy. When the tension and external pressures become too great, the system collapses and produces physical symptoms which prevent the person from continuing. There may be spasms, fainting attacks, convulsive or choreic states, and other physical symptoms. These may last until the pressure is lessened, then disappear only to return again when the tension becomes unbearable. Merely removing stress, however, is not ultimately adequate in Tarentula patients, because the primary problem is the wound-up and tense nervous system.

In the second stage of Tarentula illness, the person begins to lose control and becomes destructive. In such a state of tension, if the restless Tarentula patient is restrianed in some way, he becomes violent. At first, the destructiveness occurs only when the patient is alone. It is done in secret, hidden as much as possible from the knowledge of others. This leads to the well-known Tarentula state of fox-like cunning, and the fox-like look in the eyes.

Ultimately, however, the destructiveness becomes more uncontrolled and publicly evident. Tarentula may tear his clothes or break things. Most typically, the violence is directed at himself—self-injury, banging the head, etc—but it may also be directed at others. Stramonium also has a destructive violence, but this violence usually focuses on others and on objects, and it arises from an uncontrolled eruption from the unconscious mental levels rather than from an overly wound-up nervous system.

In the third stage of Tarentula pathology, we see two characteristic types on insanity. These may occur separately in different Tarentula patients, or at separate or alternating times within the same patient. On the one hand, there may be severe and outright violence similar to Stramonium—desire to strike and to kill, and destructive violence with superhuman strength and stamina. On the other hand, there is an erotic mania in which the person is driven to make overt sexual advances to other people, even to strangers. **Hyoscyamus** also has an erotic mania, but it is more of a passive shamelessness, rather than the active and aggressive, advances of *Tarentula*.

On the physical level, *Tarentula* has varied and profound actions on virtually every organ system. It is very much like Arsenicum in its symptomatology and modalities on the physical level. There is chilliness and great emaciation. There is also periodicity and-paroxysmal ailments. There is a profound action on the heart, with anxiety and palpitations, and mirtal valve degeneration with dyspnoea and palpitations. There are boils and carbuncles on the skin, particularly on the back between and on the scapulae. The genital organs are powerfully affected. In the female, there are fibroids, menorrhagia and nymphomania, with extreme itching of the vulva and high into the vagina. In the male, there is also great sexual desire, with pains and tumours in the testicles.

THUJA OCCIDENTALIS (*thuj.*)

It is difficult to find precise words to describe the *Thuja* state. We must resort to poetic descriptions. When you first meet a Thuja-patient you sense something which makes you cautious. He or she is very slow to trust others, and you have the feeling that he does not portray truthfully who he really is inside. Of course, everyone withholds information to some degree, but in Thuja you sense that there is more than the usual secretiveness. More than that, you have the feeling that what is being withheld is ugly—not pleasant to bring to view, either to the patient or to the prescriber. The closest we can come to describing the Thuja patient is by the words UGLY and DECEIT.

A Thuja patient is sneaky and manipulative. He or she will purposely withhold information just to test you, to see if you know what you are doing. For example, a woman has a fainting spell; she says, "I felt my soul leaving me, and I was afraid I was going to die." She gives some more information, but she does not tell you that she ate a lot of heavy food the day before. She asks, "Do you think it could be my stomach?" Having no information to suggest this possibility, you say, "No, it was more likely a drop in blood pressure." Only then does she volunteer, "But yesterday I ate a lot of heavy food!" In this way, she tries to catch you out.

Thuja patients are always reserved. They take the position of observer—they observe everything while offering nothing of themselves. They do not allow any form of deep communication. They are very closed within themselves, but not because they lack feelings. They are merely reserved and suspicious about what might happen to them if they enter into deep communication.

Thuja patients are hard people. The hardness in their emotional expression manifest even on the physical level—as hard tumours. Just so, the ugliness in their soul manifests as ugliness in the tumours.

Do not be fooled by mere appearances, however. I recall a very nice man who did very well after Thuja, but in whom it was difficult to see the Thuja essence. He was one of the nicest people one could possibly meet—very sensitive a poet. Nevertheless, he himself felt he was distant from people. He felt unable to truly communicate directly and personally, so he turned to poetry as an outlet. To see Thuja in such a case, of course, requires quite a subtle understanding of both the patient and the remedy, but once given, Thuja produces great benefit in these patients.

What exactly has the sycotic miasm done to such a patient? At first, early in the person's history, it stimulates the more base instincts. These then insist upon expression. Society, however, steps in and puts the patient "in his place". He is punished and learns to control himself. This then leads to the condition we see in Thuja. He learns to not display his real character any more, even though the tendencies remain inside and continue to cry out for expression. He finds ways to cheat. He becomes very proper. It is as if he has found out that being freely expressive of his instincts does not pay in society, so he becomes very controlled. In this way, he is tuned in to the opinions of others, but it is not a matter of being afraid of what others think, as in *Lycopodium*. In *Thuja*, it is a coldly calculated choice, for practical reasons only.

The dullness and forgetfulness eventually progresses into a despondence and dissatisfaction which can be quite deep. This is not as severe as in Nitric acid, which is also very dissatisfied, but specifically over issues of health. Thuja may have anxiety about health, but will face the problem directly. These patients are dissatisfied and despondent, but they are also cold, calculating, manipulative and scheming. They have cut themselves off. You can never know what is in their minds.

For this reason, the symptomatology in Thuja is usually UNCLEAR. You feel there is something there which you cannot quite grasp. Consequently, it is rare that you feel fully confident of a Thuja prescription. The full image is never clear because the patient never opens up enough.

As the mental pathology progresses, they develop fixed ideas. These may take different forms. Most strikingly, they describe a feeling that their legs are breakable. Kent says that their legs feel as if they are made of glass. In my experience, patients nowadays rarely say this directly. They usually describe a sensation

Thuja Occidentalis

of fragility, as if their legs are easily breakable. Actually, this is more than a mere sensation to Thuja patients.

Another strange idea they describe is that something is alive in the abdomen. They may go so far as to give elaborately exact descriptions of this feeling, it is so powerful for them. One patient said he felt a small boy inside kicking with the right foot.

Still another fixed idea that I have seen quite frequently in Thuja is the sensation that someone is walking alongside him. This is not a fear, but a delusion. By contrast, *Medorrhinum* has a FEAR that someone is behind him. Petroleum is close to *Thuja* in this regard; it has the sensation that someone else is in bed beside him.

On the physical level, as mentioned, there are all kinds of overgrowths of tissue. The tendency to warts, of course, is well-known in Thuja. In addition there may be recurrent herpes on the genitals. Women have uterine fibroids (Calc. flour., Calc. carb., Phosphorus). Fingernails and toenails are ugly and deformed.

A few keynotes should be mentioned. perspiration in Thuja has a sweetish smell. There is also a particular intolerance to onions— as well as to pungent foods in general to some degree. A rare and peculiar symptoms which I have seen only twice is running of the nose during stool.

There is a strong tendency to catarrhs of all kinds—leucorrhoea, nasal, urethral etc. The discharges themselves offer few distinguishing characteristics, but the patient in general feels relieved whenever the discharge is present.

The headaches are of a particular type. They usually begin in the forehead usually over the left eye, and then sweep back over the side of the head to the occiput. This can happen on either side, but on the right side it may be either Thuja or Prunus. (If it sweeps the right side and settles specifically on the right occipital protruberance, however, the remedy would more likely be Sanguinaria.)

Being a sycotic remedy, *Thuja* is strongly affected by wet weather. It has all kinds of rheumatic affections. It should be pointed out however, that Thuja is not very effective in the acute stage of gonorrhoea. It is more indicated once gonorrhoea has been suppressed into a deeper, chronic state. For acute gonorrhoea, better remedies to consider are *Medorrhinum, Cannabis sativa* or *Indica., Sasparilla,* and many others. If a gonorrhoea has been suppressed with antibiotics, and the patient develops warts, or worse, a chronic cachexia with diminished mental powers, be sure to think of Thuja.

Thuja also has the typical sycotic instability, but not quite in the same manner as *Medorrhinum*. The Thuja man may be quite proper, courteous and upright at the office, but he becomes an altogether different person at home. In reality, he is putting on a false facade at the office, but he has enough control to maintain it. Medorrhinum, by contrast, is not so controlled; a Medorrhinum person will tend to explode at any moment. Thuja maintains an upright, respectable facade, whereas *Medorrhinum* can be considred more a "common man".

In this sense, Thuja actually represents a deeper stage of pathology. This can be seen as well when the sycotic trait is transmitted to the next generation. Thuja is much more commonly indicated in wasted children of sycotic parents. Medorrhinum is more likely to be indicated when gonorrhoea is found in the past history of the patient himself.

The Thuja patient is more deeply sick than Medorrhinum. The idea that their legs are easily breakable is a good image for the health of the Thuja patient in general. It is a very fragile condition, on the verge of breaking down completely after just a slight push.

It is somewhat difficult to provide a good explanation for Thuja's usefulness after adverse effects from smallpox vaccinations. Such specific prescribing is ordinarily a distinct departure from the laws of cure. However, this is one exception I can confirm in my own experience. First, let me caution the reader that this only applies to smallpox vaccinations; it does not apply to other immunisations despite what Kent indicates. I believe that this is because of a resonance between the smallpox vaccination and Thuja. In other words, a patient who is very susceptible to smallpox vaccination, is also likely to be sensitive to Thuja. The pustules and vesicles common in smallpox are also found in Thuja symptomatology. The theme of ugliness also applies, because smallpox commonly leaves ugly scars (as does vaccination itself). The problem appears to be that provings alone cannot provide us with all the phases of particular medicines, hence the precise relation-

Thuja Occidentalis

ship between smallpox vaccinations and Thuja is not known.

In every medicine, there is always a sequence of events. Pathology begins somewhere and ends somewhere. To fully know a remedy, we must know each stage very clearly. The same remedy will act both in the beginning phases and in the end stages. For example, if you have a patient with chronic headaches dating from a smallpox vaccination, *Thuja* will likely cure them even though they may not fit the typical left-sided frontal headaches of Thuja. For this to happen, the patient must be in a phase not yet elucidated in the provings.

This is why we sometimes must rely heavily on the causative factor in a case. We know that smallpox can cause maningitis, an ailment characterised by the most violent of headaches. Nevertheless, it is important to specify that *Thuja* will bring about cure on such specific causative indications OFTEN—but by no means ALWAYS. One must always take the full case to determine if another remedy covers the case adequately. If not, then one is justified to use Thuja.

Another ROUTINE use of *Thuja* is in warts which have been suppressed. Here it is appropriate to THINK of Thuja. Caution is again in order, however, because I can testify from personal experience to several mistakes made by just such routine use of Thuja.

Thuja is a very deep acting remedy that can produce some amazing surprises. You may come to a point of desperation in a case. No progress has been made after several prescriptions. The patient is very closed, proper, and correct—you may even think of Kali carb. but it doesn't work. Finally, you realise that the patient is not really being straight with you; there is this manipulative deviousness. Once you see this, you give Thuja, and you are likely to see dramatic benefits indeed.

TUBERCULINUM BOVINUM KENT
(*tub.*

Tuberculinum is a distinctive remedy which cannot be missed once it is understood, but one which is difficult to describe concisely. Tuberculinum patients can be unpredictable in their moods and behaviour. One minute they are refined and gentle; the next, malicious and destructive.

Inside, Tuberculinum patients are people who burn the candle at both ends. They feel that life is short and must be lived to the fullest. They are never truly satisfied with themselves, nor with other people. They tend to be people with much ability and vitality in the early stages but they do not conserve themselves. They dissipate themselves. They are full of contradictory feelings; on the one hand they seek fulfillment and change, and on the other they feel dissatisfied and irritable.

For example, consider the Tuberculinum child. He can never be satisfied by anything—like Cina or Chamomilla. It is more than a momentary impulsive capriciousness in Tuberculinum, however. It is a deep dissatisfaction which leads to destructiveness. The Tuberculinum child is intentionally malicious. He will find out what your most prized possession is and he will break it (see Breaks Things in Repertory). Just when you are about to go somewhere, he will throw an uncontrollable tantrum just to spoil your plans. He will do exactly that he has been told not to do merely to be spiteful. He may swear at his mother. Inside, he may wonder why he does these things, but he cannot control himself. Tuberculinum children become a constant torment to their parents. They are capable of disrupting entire families.

A similar pathology manifests in the adult. He is dissatisfied. He doesn't know what he really wants, and no-one else can find ways of satisfying him. He becomes irritable over daily circumstances and he flies to pieces. He swears at his wife on no account. He cannot help himself.

Tuberculinum patients are difficult people to live with. They are aggressive and malicious. They are exceptionally selfish. They seek self-gratification, but they never achieve it.

In their dissatisfaction, Tuberculinum patients continuallly seek change. They go from job to job, or from location to location—always seeking escape from their dilemmas. Once they make a change, they may at first feel contented, but soon they again become dissatisfied and want to move on. These are people described in the books as being "cosmpolitan"—but this is a pathological cosmopolitanism. They not only have a desire for travel; they are DRIVEN to it.

People who have had clinical experience with tubercular patients, will have little difficulty grasping the Tuberculinum picture. These are patients who are lean, quick, muscular—like Sulphur, Phosphorus, Nux vomica. They have rapid metabolisms and burn fat quickly. They emaciate quickly; once the disease has taken hold, they progress rapidly toward destruction and death. The Tuberculinum patient, even without necessarily having the disease, carries this feeling of death and destruction deep inside. He feels his life is going to be short, so he hastens to make the most of it while he can.

Sexually, tubercular patients are known to be hyperactive. Just so, Tuberculinum patients have strong sexual desire. They go from one relationship to another, but always their love affairs are tumultuous. There are many upheavals and conflicts. In their capriciousness and need for change they are difficult to understand or to please.

Clinical experience has shown that tubercular patients heal better in mountain forests with dry climate. This is true for Tuberculinum patients as well. If they feel irritated, they usually want to be alone, and the best thing for them to do is to walk in the open air in the mountains. For some reason, they are particularly ameliorated by being in pine forests. Conversely, they do not feel well at the seashore. In general, they are aggravated by cold wet weather and ameliorated in warm dry climates.

Tuberculinum patients, because their metabolisms burn fat so readily, have a desire for fat. Especially they desire pork and pungent-tasting meats like salami and smoked meats. They also have a desire for ice-cream.

Of course, Tuberculinum patients perspire heavily, particularly at night. This is a profuse perspiration all over the body, drenching the bedclothes. They may have to get up during the night to change their night clothes. This is not a particularly offensive perspiration, and it may not be accompanied by fever.'

A characteristic keynote of Tuberculinum is fear of dogs and cats—especially the latter. The fear of cats alone may often lead you to Tuberculinum in difficult cases. Sometimes this is not described as a fear but rather a disgust. They say they hate cats; they cannot stand to touch cats. They may even have allergies to the fur of cats or dogs.

The destructiveness of Tuberculinum is manifest in another keynote symptom. I have observed in cured cases; if they see a sharp knife they imagine the noise it would make if plunged into someone—the crunching of bones and tissues.

Although *Tuberculinum* should never be prescribed routinely, it nevertheless is often indicated in patients with a personal history or family history of tuberculosis. Once such a history is uncovered in a case, it is always worth-while to inquire about other keynotes—fear of cats, desire for pork, desire for fat, heavy perspiration, frequent colds, maliciousness, desire for change, etc. If the confirmatory picture is present, one is then justified to prescribe Tuberculinum.

Often we see patients who have had tuberculosis in the past, but have been treated by antibiotics. If they have been treated with Streptomycin there may occur a crippling vertigo. It is a vertigo which is not specific; there are no modalities. It seems to these patients as if the head is cramped, or as if it is full of rubbish. This symptomatology may respond to Tuberculinum, but we may some day discover that potentised Streptomycin will display this symptom in its provings.

VERATRUM ALBUM (*verat.*)

The Veratrum influence is constant activity. This is not so much violence or aggressiveness, except in the most extreme state. It is rather a driven, ceaseless energy compelling the patient to be busy all the time. It is likely to be activity for its own sake, without purpose—constantly stacking books or chairs, endless cleaning. In the hyperactive child, it is unceasing drawing, painting, singing, playing, but unlike Stramonium, it is not breaking things or destructive. Such a person may be a pest, demanding attention by sheer energy, but not actually destructive.

The Veratrum patient has a profound confusion about his identity. He thinks he is Christ or John the Baptist, or a chosen person sent to save the world. This is the street corner preacher who, day in and day out, exhorts people to repent, repeating over and over the same righteous message, often at the top of his lungs. Unlike Stramonium, the actual physical strength is not increased, but rather there is surprising stamina. The person seems never to run out of steam. In Stramonium, we see an eruption of the unconscious, and the person may experience a wide variety of delusions about what is happening to him. In Veratrum, the person does not SEE delusions so much as he has a mistaken idea of his own identity. He is convinced of who he is, and no-one can talk him out of it. It is as if the organism sidetracked the energy rising from the unconscious into a relatively more harmless confusion of identity.

In the most early stages, the ceaseless activity, singing, doing repetitive tasks etc. may be difficult to distinguish from other remedies. The Veratrum quality becomes clear a little later, when the person exhibits righteousness. This may not yet have religious content to it, but the person will believe himself to be superior to those around him. He may become overly critical, censorious. In the Repertory, we see Veratrum is in bold type under the rubric HAUGHTY. As this tendency grows, the person becomes less in touch with the discrepancy between his reality and others; he may believe himself to be the only one who is sane, all the others being insane. Finally, this develops the full religious righteousness.

The active state may alternate with a melancholy state—as in some manic depressive psychoses. The patient may brood or sulk, despairing over his own state or over the state of the world. In particular, there is despair over his own salvation. In young girls, just before the menses, there may be a deep despair, particularly if there is dysmenorrhoea with coldness, prostration, sweating, vomiting and/or diarrhoea. This despair, over the years, may progress into a full-fledged insanity of the Veratrum type.

Some of the general characteristics of *Veratrum* are distinctive, and helpful in prescribing. *Veratrum* has great thirst for cold drinks, even for ice. It also desires fruit, particularly acid fruit. There is a great desire for salt. And throughout the Veratrum state there is severe coldness.

The acute state of Veratrum shows the activity in exaggerated form once again, both mentally and physically. The excessive vomiting and diarrhoea is very active, sudden, explosive. The classic Vertrum state is one of severe illness, even shock. The best description is found in Kent's Materia Medica; "Profuse watery" discharges. These conditions occur without apparent provocation. In cholera or cholera morbus, it seems that the fluids are forced out of the body. Lies in bed, relaxed prostrated, cold to the fingertips, with corresponding blueness, fairly purple; lips cold and blue, countenance pinched and shrunken; great sensation of coldness as if the blood were ice-water; scalp cold; forehead covered with cold sweat; headache and exhaustion; coldness in spots over the body; extremities cold as death. Full of cramps; looks as if he would die. This state comes out during the menses, during colic with nausea, with mania and violent delirium, with headache, with violent inflammations.

In the muscles, there is much twitching (like Hyoscyamus and Agaricus).

Physically, other than the gastrointestinal and menstrual symptoms, there are severe neualgic pains which drive the person to mania. There are severe neuralgic pains in the head, as well as congestive pains in the head. In the extremities and joints, there are severe neuralgic and rheumatic pains, again causing mania, coldness, and sweat.

In comparison, *Veratrum* is highly active like *Stramonium* and *Tarentula* more so than *Hyoscyamus*. It is not so violent or so threatening as are *Stramonium* or *Tarentula*. Of course, in the most extreme states, it can be violent, but this is not characteristic of the full course of the illness. It is more religious, righteous, censorious, and haughty than the other remedies.

INDEX OF REMEDIES

A
Aconitum napellus	11, 35, 80, 85
Aesculus hippocastanum	52
Aethusa cynapium	1, 57
Agaricus muscarius	2, 87, 148, 167, 212
Agnus castus	3, 4, 11, 51
Allium Cepa	115
Alumina	5-9, 56, 119-121, 165, 168, 169, 178
Ambra grisea	12
Anacardium orientale	107, 164
Apis mellifica	53, 62, 91, 171
Argentum nitricum	10-12, 56, 77
Arnica montana	26, 59
Arsenicum album	2, 7, **14**-20, 33, 34, 48-50, 61-63, 71, 94, 114, 115, 124, 139, 144, 147, 158, 159, 163, 173, 179, 184, 199, 201, 202
Asafoetida	131
Asarum europaeum	148
Aurum foliatum	**21**-25, 100, 151, 188, 200

B
Baptisia tinctoria	124
Baryta carbonica	**26**-28, 93
Baryta muriatica	29, 181
Belladonna	34, 35, 85, 87, 98, 106, 195, 196
Bismuthum subnitricum	**30**, 31
Bovista lycoperdon	53
Bryonia	**32**-36, 80, 106, 184

C
Calcarea corbonica	12, 17, 26, 28, 33, **37**-43, 52, 53, 61, 68, 69, 71, 74, 75, 77, 106, 112, 125, 139, 160, 178, 180, 181-184, 205
Calcarea fluorica naturalis	181, 205
Calcarea phosphorica	**42**-46, 57, 154, 172

Index of Remedies

	Calcarea sulphurica	82, 142
	Calcarea Silicata	142
	Cannabis india	2, **47-51**, 106, 162, 205
	Cannabis sativa	205
	Capsicum	**52**
	Carbo animalis	**61**
	Carbo vegetabilis	52, **59-63**
	Carcinosinum Burnett	73
	Causticum Hahnemanni	**54-58**, 90, 148, 160, 197, 198
	Chamomilla	35, 44, 53, 79, 115, 208
	Chelidonium majus	61, **64-67**
	Cimicifuga racemosa	45, 172
	Cina	53, 208
	Cistus canadensis	122, 173
	Clematis erecta	24
	Cocculus indicus	8, 165
	Coffea cruda	160, 191
	Conium maculatum	12
D	Dulcamara	64, **68-71**
F	Ferrum metallicum	52, 77, 170, 183
	Fluoricum acidum	**72-73**
	Formica rufa	35
G	Gelsemium sempervirens	35, 80, 111, 152, 179
	Graphites naturalis	9, 58, **74-78**, 158, 181
	Gratiola officinalis	79
	Grindelia robusta	1
H	Helleborus niger	53
	Helonias dioica	124, 152, 184
	Hepar sulphuris calcareum	13, 26, 61, **80-82**, 148
	Hydrophobinum see Lyssin	
	Hyoscyamus niger	**85-87**, 93, 106, 148, 164, 196, 202, 212
I	Ignatia amara	1, 46, **88-89**, **91-93**, 122, 124, 135,

		136, 150, 152, 162, 171, 173, 177, 179, 187-189
K	Kali arsenicosum	2, 18, 94
	Kali bichromicum	52, 53, **94**-98, 115, 182
	Kali bromatum	106
	Kali carbonicum	18, 21, 68, 71, 98, **99**-104, 172, 182
	Kali iodatum	115
	Kreosotum	57
L	Lac caninum	57
	Lachesis muta	1, 49, 60, 61, 93, 102, **105**-107, 120, 158, 160, 168, 171, 175, 179, 185
	Ledum palustre	121
	Lilium tigrinum	89, 131, 136
	Lycopodium clavatum	9, 18, 62, 64, 66, 67, 102, **108**, 112, 121, 137, 147, 192, 204
	Lyssinum (Hydrophobinum)	83
M	Magnesia carbonica	116
	Magnesia phosphorica	115
	Magnesia muriatica	**113**-116
	Mancinella	106
	Medorrhinum	9, 22, 57, 90, 115, **117**-122, 205, 206
	Mercurius solubilis	7, 9, 52, **123**-129, 135, 153, 163, 165
	Mezereum	101, 135
	Moschus	89, 131, 136, 168
	Muriaticum acidum	150, 152-154, 185, 186
N	Natrum carbonicum	52, 133,
	Natrum muriaticum	15, 16, 21, 26, 35, 52, 58, 75, 88, 89, 91, 93, 106, 112, 125, **130**-137, 150, 160, 162, 171, 178, 179, 185, 188, 189, 200
	Natrum sulphuricum	76, 133, 173
	Nitric acidum	2, 13, 17, 18, 48, 82, 102, **138**-

	Nux moschata	142, 181, 182, 204
		35
	Nux vomica	15, 20, 53, 62, 73, 79, 81, 82, 93, 102, 104, 177, 122, 125, 126, **143**-149, 160, 163, 177, 193, 199, 209
O	Opium	186
	Origanum majorana	105, 160
P	Petroleum	205
	Phosphoricum acidum	43, 51, 52, 59, 88, 92, 95, 100, 120, 125, **150**-154, 175, 185
	Phosphorus	2, 14-19, 30, 31, 34, 41, 44, 45, 48, 49, 63, 69, 74, 77, 89, 90, 93, 102, 104, 115, 125, 135, 136, 144, 153, **155**-159, 165, 168, 170, 171, 172, 177, 179, 197, 205, 209
	Picricum acidum	150, 153, 154
	Platinum metallicum	7, 79, 90, 105, 106, 126, 147, **160**-164
	Plumbum metallicum	**165**-169
	Prunus spinosa	205
	Psorinum	181
	Pulsatilla pratensis	28, 62, 77, 90, 96, 121, 122, 135, 136, 150, 153, **170**-173, 179, 181, 182, 183
R	Rhododendron chrysanthum	24, 62
	Rhus toxicodendron	12, 34, 45, 58, 68, 96, 114, 115, 172, 173
S	Sabadilla	162
	Sanguinaria canadensis	205
	Sanicula aqua	115
	Sarsaparilla	205
	Secale cornutum	12, 62
	Sepia	22, 58, 81, 82, 90, 91, 137, 150, 151, 160, 172, **174**-178
	Silicea terra (=Silica)	9, 112, 168, **179**-182, 184, 198

	Spigelia anthelmia	106
	Stannum metallicum	124, **183-186**
	Staphysagria	54, 73, 105, 113, 160, 162, 179, **187-192**
	Stramonium	12, 86, 87, 106, 117, 191, **193-196**, 201, 211, 213
	Sulphuricum acidum	80, 125, 199
	Sulphur lotum	9, 19, 73, 91, 102, 135, 170, 181, 209
	Syphilinum	127, **197**, 198
T	*Tarentula hispanica*	26, 106, 117, 119, 122, 125, 164, 195, 196, **199-202**, 213
	Thuja occidentalis	57, 122, **203-207**
	Tuberculinum bovinum Kent	9, 28, 44, 157, **208-210**
V	*Valeriana officinalis*	89
	Veratrum album	61, 87, 106, 164, 196, 200, **211-213**
Z	*Zincum metallicum*	12, 167